There's No Food in Your Food™

Should You Strip Paint with it or Feed it to Your Children?

To speak to the Authors or schedule a Class: 18632897263

Email: Miriam@vigoacuisine.com

Kristi@vigoacuisine.com

Get the first book Shake, Splash & Eat! Shockingly Simple Recipes on the website www.vigoacuisine.com

www.Facebook.com/VigoaCuisine

www.Instagram.com/CanaryIslandOliveOil

www.VigoaCuisine.Wordpress.com (the Blog)

www.VigoaCuisine.Etsy.com (NEW Site)

www.twitter.com/kristilinebaugh

www.twitter.com/miriamvigoa

Printed in the United States of America

TABLE OF CONTENTS

Chapter 1

The Sausage Fingers Epidemic
In this chapter we will share the secret reason you may be suffering with Sausage Fingers and Cankles.

Now, let's be clear. This book is Not about everyone losing weight because we all need to look like J.J. Virgin. Although she looks amazing, very amazing, I have at this point in my life become comfortable with the idea of being healthy first and the weightloss being an agreeable side-effect.

(So now you can relax and enjoy the read, no soap box seats required!)

Why is it, when you eat sometimes you feel just fine, and others you feel like your stomach pulled a rip cord on a life raft exploding inside you? You can forget catching your breath.

Why in the World? Do you wake up, your hands and feet aching like you got run over by a mob of ironman triathletes?

No! Not again. Yesterday, you woke up, bright eyed and bushy tailed, and today you wake up, eyes so puffy and swollen you look like you went 3 rounds with a 700 lb gorilla? (And lost!)

How does this happen? Going out with friends, you grab your favorite dress shoes, your feet are so swollen, it would take a miracle to squish on your favorite slip-ons.

Why me? It's a guessing game. When you eat, you suddenly have horrific gas, bloating and have to run for your life to the bathroom with diarrhea?

Why is that?

True story. I remember since I was a small child, I always had a "funny stomach". I still can feel the embarrassment of my Mom writing a note to my teacher telling her I needed to take my pink pills. I crumbled the note up on the walk to school and threw it along with the Pepto Bismol tabs, in the ditch. Boy I wished I had never done that. Isn't it crazy that a "funny stomach" can be so horrifying?

I had attacks of diarrhea so severe, I still remember the fateful day of "the accident." I will spare you the gooey details, I'm sure you can imagine. Or maybe, like me, you've had a "not so funny stomach" all your life. Finally after a lifetime, of "shit'uations" we have answers.

You may not believe us, and I can understand why.

 Most of the time, problems that have plagued, hounded and tormented us and our family for years feel like they have to have, must have , a very long complicated process for annihilation. Problems that have been such an intimate part of our genetics are surely inherited, every magical potion we tried, has failed. The answer must be out of reach, out of our control out of our understanding.

The Answer

Is Ridiculously simple and it's hiding in plain sight: You have been suffering from "sodium and chemical overload", putting your body in a lethal fight with a deadly predator.

 The Undeniable Truth is. There's No Food in Your Food!

Have you ever had Sausage Fingers?

Technically it's called Edema. Which is slang for, "Oh My God! My fingers are swollen up like little fat sausage fingers, I can't get my rings off."

How does that happen? You go out to eat, order a meal or split an appetizer eat your soup and salad, go home and wake up in the morning with "Sausage Fingers".

The culprit? The restaurant meal had 3,000 to 5,000mg of sodium in it.

No way you say ;-) "How is that even possible, nobody uses that much salt." Well unfortunately it's because everything is processes pre-seasoned and dipped dunked fried or marinated in salt-packed sauces and hydrogenated oils.

Imagine a family table filled with food you would have eaten for three whole days, see the bigness of that, now look at the serving you had for dinner. Three days of salt at once is why you have "sausage fingers".

Typically Sausage Fingers is not on the Menu, but you will be taking some home!

The days when Grandma fixed one chicken for all six of us, are sadly gone. I remember my Grandma had one chicken and lots of veggies and salad and homemade bread, cucumber and onions. It was totally acceptable for the kids to have one chicken leg and the rest of the plate was filled with sides.

My Grandma would laugh and say, "thank goodness there are only two kids here today because they don't make 3 legged chickens."

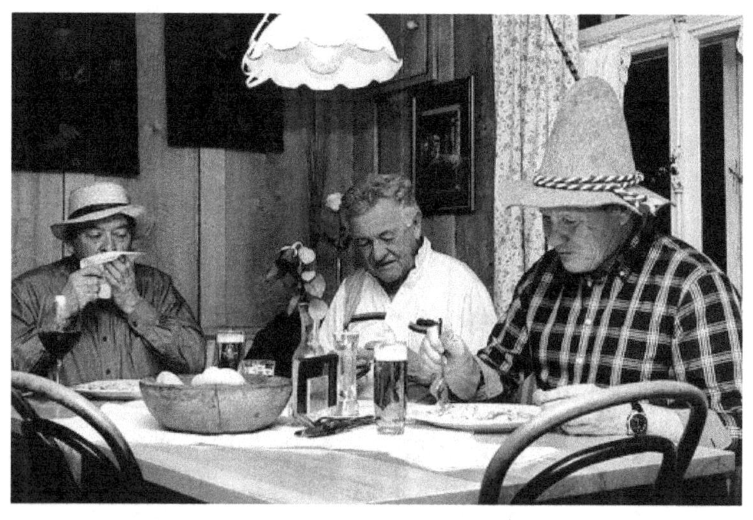

Health Tip By the way, American Heart Association recommends 1,500 a day. So that restaurant outing just cost you over 3x's the recommended allowance.

We have all suffered the effects of high salt diets. Even though we didn't realize that was the problem.

Miriam: You know I want to stop right here and interject something I have heard so many people say at our classes and shows. We have done hundreds of shows and have spoken to tens of thousands of people. So many people are under the impression that if they themselves don't use salt, they won't have any salt related health issues.

I just left a supermarket I usually pay extra for rotisserie chicken without chemicals and sodium. They were sold out. Doesn't that tell us more people are buying chemical free? I was reading the ingredients of regular chicken, it had 10% sodium solution injected in it and MSG listed 3 times. Two of the other ones I remember, maltodextrin and dextrose which are added to flavor and preserve.

It is no wonder people walk around with sacks of fluid under their eyes and swollen ankles. Never mind the headaches and other ill effects.

Kroger has a chicken called Simple Truth that uses chicken, water and sea salt. That one seems to be very good. Whole Foods has one that is called Naked that looks good too.

Kristi: I know what you mean. The other day at a show a customer told me he was forced to be on a low sodium diet, his kidneys were failing, he was shocked how much salt is in food that wouldn't seem it would have salt in it. Even low sodium items have too much salt he said. Like cereal and bread, can be loaded with salt.

Edema from overloading salt doesn't just give you Sausage Fingers, it gives you Cankles.

Kristi: A student came to our cooking class, looking for a chair to prop her feet up during the class. It was a bit awkward for her, she wanted to be in front but didn't want to prop her feet in front of everybody. She got situated in front, we always have great people, nobody cared if she propped her feet up. She said her Cankles were bothering her.

We asked her what Cankles were, she said, "I have been eating out a lot lately, there is so much salt in the food that it makes my ankle swell up to match the size of my calf. Cankle.

Everybody laughed. It is a funny name. The pain behind her eyes couldn't totally be covered by the laughter.

We always spend time with our students after a class answering questions, especially when things like that come up, we want to give them hope that it doesn't have to be that way forever.

Miriam: It makes my heart smile when we can coach a student on techniques to have restaurant flavor at home and not feel like they have to eat out all the time.

Kristi: I remember that student after you talked with her she said she really felt she had a chance to change her eating.

How many times have you eaten at a restaurant and the next morning your eyes are swollen and puffy and you just don't "feel right". Or 20 minutes later or even later that evening you have a massive attack of diarrhea.

It's not "just how you are". It's all the chemicals and salt your body is desperately trying to flush out. We do it so often it's "just how it is", or "Well, that's part of aging", baggy, saggy eyes and swollen achy joints.

Warning

Attention Diabetics: If you are eating foods that give you diarrhea, you are negatively affecting your blood sugar!

When food is rushed through your system, (technically it's called, dumping syndrome), like it is when you have diarrhea, it puts too much sugar in your system at once and your sugar will spike. Not what our Diabetic customers want to hear, I'm afraid.

Kristi: It doesn't pick convenient times I'm afraid. When it hits you suddenly, you are subject to many an uninvited "adventure".

Actually this outhouse reminds me of an unitived adventure I took up in the mountains of Vermont, all was quiet in the forest just me the footpath packed with soggy leaves and the wild chipmunk that insisted I had a grape hidden somewhere in my pocket! At least that's what the owner of the hunting camp told me when both the chipmunk and I came in from the outhouse hike!

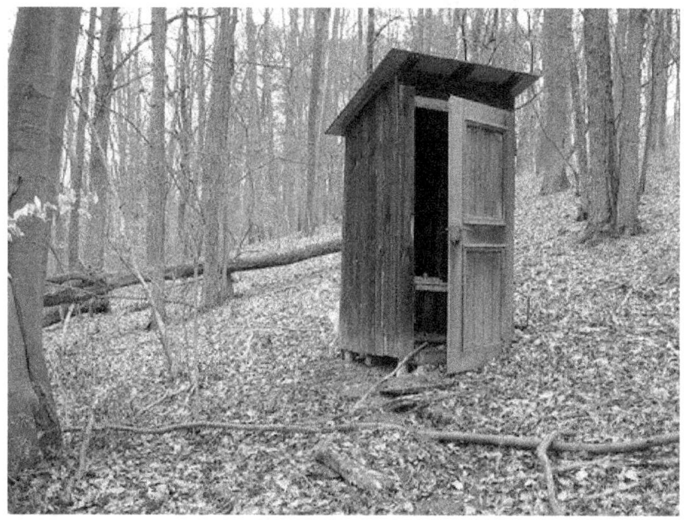

Come to think of it, the chipmunk got a grape, I never did. ;-)

Miriam: While we are still on topic speaking of Diabetics. I speak to a lot of people who suffer with diabetes and always hear what a battle it is to find things to eat. Everybody wants a treat now and then whether dessert or other goodie. There is an entire industry of sugar free products. Have you eaten a lot of sugar free stuff in your search to lose weight?

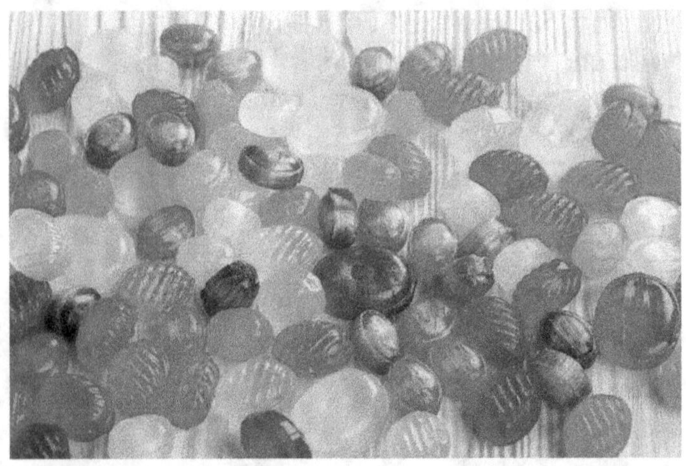

Kristi: Oh my God yes! I have eaten every kind of sugar free candy, cake, ice cream, soda and cookie that ever was created. I wanted the sweet but not the sugar. I had many an effect that you just spoke of, cramping and diarrhea like a fire hose.

Miriam: Well that's a visual, I'll not soon forget.

Kristi: I know right? Talking about dumping syndrome, I remember one horrific day, actually the last time I ever ate sugar free candy, to think about it, anything sugar free. I had eaten a bag of sugar free candy. I was at home Thank God.

 I was on the toilet, doubled over, screaming from the cramps and the pain, I was praying for God to take away the Pain. I couldn't breathe and I was crying and sweating. The pain would wash over me nearly drowning me I would catch enough breath to keep from passing out. It was probably thirty minutes before I could slowly drag myself off the toilet and crawl to bed. I will never forget that.

Miriam: How scary. It is really sad to think manufacturers continue to put things in our food that not only have effects like that, but are marketing to people who already have a compromised system and are struggling with diabetes. Or food that is geared toward fat free or calorie free for dieters.

If there is No Fat, No Calories, No Carbs in your Food...Then there's also No Food in your Food.

Kristi: An interesting note to diabetics, a lot of the sugar free candies and cookies and desserts have a warning that the sugar substitutes used will give you diarrhea if you eat too much. Isn't that odd? Here eat this and it will spike your sugar then pump in more insulin to bring it down. An ugly cycle.

Miriam: Just imagine if you wouldn't have realized that it was the sugar free candy that caused the attack. You could have been taken to the hospital that would have spiraled into a whole new level of drama.

How many times do people mistake dumping syndrome for irritable bowel syndrome?

Miriam: That is so true, I have a friend who was diagnosed with IBS and she suffers horribly. The symptoms from the www.aboutibs.org website lists the symptoms as follows.

"The essential feature of IBS is abdominal pain …. the pain is associated with a change in bowel habit. This means that the frequency or consistency of stools–either diarrhea or constipation–changes when the pain occurs."

The symptoms come and go and vary from constipation to diarrhea with bloating and pain.

Kristi: Sounds more like my attack could have been called, Irritable Sugar Free Candy Syndrome. I wonder how many people are just reacting to the food but are being diagnosed as irritable bowel syndrome.

Kristi: True story. Many years ago in college, no we won't say how long ago! I was diagnosed with irritable bowel syndrome. I was going through a major loss in my life I was emotionally eating. Have you ever done that?

Miriam: Of course. I'm sure most everyone has.

Kristi: I told them I didn't have it but they said "young ladies my age" often have it because of all the stress in college. Looking back more likely it came from the fact that we were away from home for the first time and eating pizza, hot dogs, ice cream, mountain dew, honey buns and ramen ... for breakfast!

I had "Sausage Fingers" constantly in college, so bad in fact that in the morning I couldn't bend my fingers at the middle joint without the joint popping in and out.

Miriam: How painful. Isn't it amazing that we all want to jump on the "let's go to the Doctor" bus and run off to get a pill to fix it. I'm surprised they didn't tell you that you had arthritis.

Kristi: They did, how funny you said that. They wanted to test me for rheumatoid arthritis.

Recap:

Sausage Fingers are Not normal. Like puffy bags under your eyes. It's not "Just How You Are."

Irritable Bowel syndrome may be just what it says. Irritable, so stop putting stuff in there to aggravate it. ;-)

If you eat a "food" that is sugar free, fat free, no calories, then there is no Food either. Because food has calories and fat because it's what our bodies need to survive.

Food, it's what Feeds you.

So basically, if you are reading a salad dressing bottle and it says no calories ... mmmh that can't be right. Right?

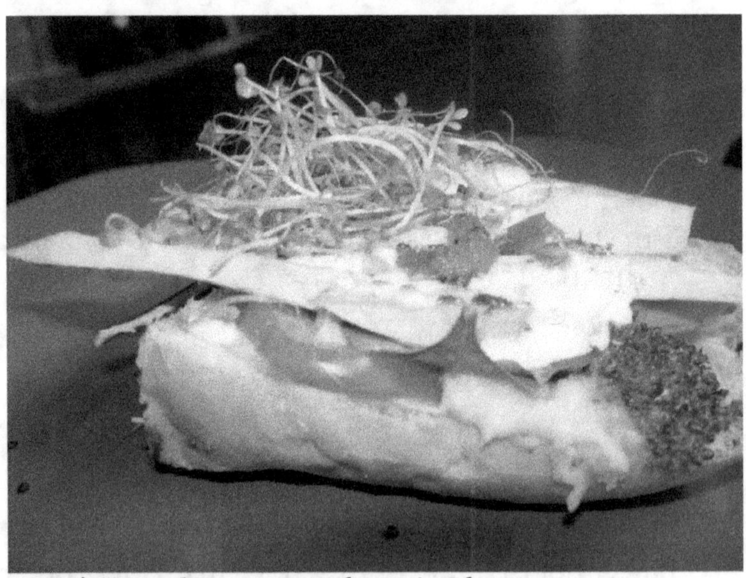

Here's a real customer favorite from our restaurant.

Open Face Hummus and Avocado Sandwich

It has radish sprouts but you can use broccoli sprouts or bean sprouts whichever is more accessible. The radish sprouts have a bit of a spicy finish which goes really well with the Lime Canary Island Garlic Herb Olive Oil. We drizzled it over the fresh veggies, a little fresh mozzarella and shazam that's some good eatin!

You can easily turn it into a panini just leave off the sprouts until after your have pressed it. Add a little Splash to the top of the bread before you press it. The herbs get nice and crunchy.

www.hopefoods.com is a great new Hummus Miriam found for us while doing shows in Traverse City Michigan so we put it on everything while we were up there. I think I saw it at Lucky's Market down in Florida.

 I am totally in Love with this brand of hummus. 1 Gram of protein per 2 Tablespoons I like it with other protein foods like broccoli, cauliflower and Ryvita crackers.

 We also love the company because they are persnickety about Fresh, Honest Ingredients, like we are. Check them out you will be Wowed!

Chapter 2

A New Disease or Last Night's Dinner?

In this chapter we discuss why the risk of having a heart attack increases 4x after having a heavy meal for dinner. Is it the size of the meal? Or something else.

So many, "ailments" can be attributed from eating gobs of processed salt and other chemicals from early morning till late night.

It's Not Your Fault.

You have a job, sometimes two, kids, pets, meetings, civic organizations, house duties, on and on. Rushing through the Drive-Thru, microwaving a frozen dinner, picking up "curbside" has become an American Habit. But it may be driving us down a long and dusty, lonely road of symptoms and diseases as hard to figure out as the remote for the new T.V.

Are you suffering from these highly diagnosed diseases? Do you notice your heart pounding or being irregular after you eat?

Miriam: I know I have heard Kristi talk about her heart doing flip flops after we eat out sometimes.

Kristi: It is crazy. There is a steak house that I don't eat at anymore because they put their "house seasoning" on everything so even if you order without it it's still all over the grill. Every time I would eat there my neck would turn red I would feel hot and my heart started doing backward flips and I couldn't breathe.

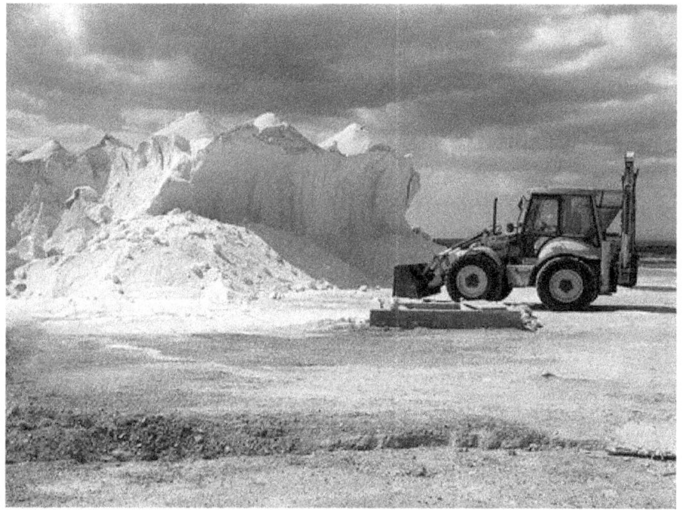

We are eating Mountains of Salt

(this is actually a pile of salt used in water softeners, so we are eating and drinking mountains of salt!)

FYI:

Irregular heartbeat has been linked to excess sodium intake

Water retention is directly linked to excess sodium.

High blood pressure can be directly linked to excess sodium and sugar.

Kidney disease is linked to high blood pressure which is linked to sodium and sugar consumption.

Stroke

Heart Failure

Osteoporosis

Stomach Cancer eating highly salted foods can double the risk for stomach cancer

Kidney Disease some cases of kidney failure can be linked to Heartburn medications (CBS News)

Enlarged Heart Muscle

Headaches

ATTENTION Women:

High blood pressure is the leading risk factor for death in women in the U.S!

 That is 400,000 Female deaths a year. That's 5x's the annual deaths from breast cancer.

Here is another mind blowing fact. Women in their 30's and 40's are experiencing a rising trend in incidents of heart attack and women 45 and older, have less of a survival chance a year after their heart attack, than male survivors.

According to The Heart Foundation. Org I was horrified to learn that as I sit here writing this and you read this in your favorite comfy chair, there will be 1 Female death every minute, imagine your living room empty now: in one hour it is filled with 60 dead bodies of your closest girlfriends piled at your feet..

Horrified? We are. We all should be.

Processed Engineered Salt is Toxic: It's NOT A Food

But I Don't use Salt! We don't even have a salt shaker on the table! There is No Way I am drowning in salt and chemicals.

Miriam: We hear that at every class, every seminar every show. The last question they usually ask is, "How did I develop heart disease, it just must be hereditary? Or diabetes, kidney disease or, you insert so many diseases.

People never suspect that it could be linked to the chemicals in the food.

Many people just blame their genetics and assume they have to die the same way everyone else in their family died.

Miriam: I tell our students just because many of your family members died of heart disease it is not sentencing you to the same fate.

Look at it as a warning, so you know that your family is sensitive in that area so be sure to take good care of your diet to avoid the same "fate."

Kristi: I always like what you tell people. "What was, doesn't have to be what is." I've learned a surprising lesson about this life we live it's not only what you are doing it's what you aren't doing.

If you aren't eating fresh foods but instead are eating packaged food.

There is a Surprise inside! You are eating more chemicals than food!

Of course there are exceptions people are born with diabetes, compromised heart or kidneys.

They aren't who we are talking about. We are talking about a perfectly normal 30 year old who suddenly has diabetes, kidney stones and ulcerative colitis. We are talking about people who suddenly have thyroid problems or are peeing on themselves.

Miriam: That reminds me of a story. I was watching T.V the other day I had the commercials on mute and happened to look up at a commercial. There were two women dancing and dancing, laughing and smiling, dancing all around. It peaked my interest I wondered if they had won a contest, they were obviously celebrating something. I turned up the volume and they were advertising a new Pee Pad.

Kristi: Pee Pad? Is that what it was called?

Miriam: No but it could have been. It was a pad that holds more urine than the other brand. These were young women, celebrating a product that will catch the urine when they pee on themselves. They make it appear fun and exciting that you can now go around and not have a problem when you pee. I think that is a Red Flag, it is Not normal for us to urinate on ourselves. If you are, we need to find an answer not a pad that holds more urine.

Kristi: That is another symptom that is minimized by a quick fix. We want people to know is, that you aren't just getting older so that is the way life is!

No! No! No!

It's not normal to have Bowel Leakage either, which they now sell pads for as well. If it's coming out in an uncontrollable way, we must look at what went in, in the first place!

Let's take a look at the Surprise Inside our food and we aren't talking about Cracker Jacks!

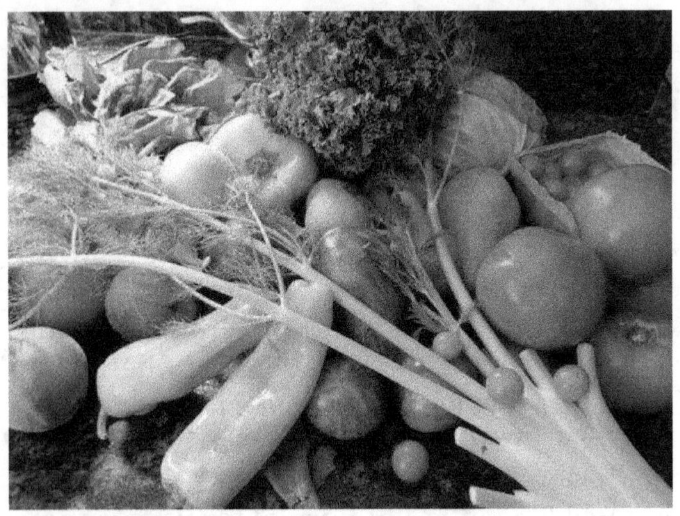

Most of us, as silly as it may seem to the manufactures, most of us assume that there is actually food in our food. So when we see the commercial for Ranch dressing we would assume there are all types of lovely veggies in there.

 I felt like a dope for buying this dip!

Take a quick Peek inside: **Ranch Dressing**

We all grew up eating Ranch dressing, I did anyway, did you? Heck we even dunked our pizza in it and sent our salads swimming in it. Poor little salad.

Ranch Dressing has 21 Ingredients

Check out all the No Food ingredients in here.

Soybean Oil, Water, Egg Yolk, Sugar, Salt, Cultured Nonfat Buttermilk, Natural Flavors (Soy), Spices. Less than 1% of Dried Garlic, Dried Onion, Vinegar, Phosphoric Acid, Xanthan Gum, Modified Food Starch, Monosodium Glutamate, Artificial Flavors, Disodium Phosphate, Sorbic Acid and Calcium Disodium EDTA as Preservatives, Disodium Inosinate and Disodium Guanylate.

ATTENTION: Did you Notice? MSG and, salt or a chemicalized version of salt is used 6 different times in the one dressing. Disodium Inosinate and Disodium Guanylate are used to increase the flavor in processed foods, along with MSG.

The first ingredient is soybean oil which is the cheapest processed oil. Soybean Oil as well as canola and grapeseed oil is processed with hexane which is a byproduct of gasoline, and is an excitotoxin and carcinogen and is used in sealants, coatings and Rust-Oleum.

That's not even getting to the rest of the meal and your body is already choking on sodium overload with chemicals. Ranch dressing is the number one selling salad dressing on the market. We have heard countless parents say the only way to get their kids to eat veggies is give them ranch dressing to dunk the veggies in.

Eye-opening Fact

Ranch dressing has Titanium Dioxide in it to make it white. So does Sunscreen and Paint.

"Do you strip paint with it or feed it to your Children?"

I was pretty freaked out to see blue yogurt, apples that taste like grapes. Yes they make apples to taste like a grape by soaking it in Methyl Anthranilate an artificial grape flavor to make the skin taste grape.

Gatorade full of artificial colors and high fructose corn syrup. Cereals with Superhero characters and a list of ingredients as tall as you're 4 year old.

Miriam: The brighter side of this conversation is that the kids don't usually have a debit card when they are under 13 years old. So we really do have the power to keep their chemical loads under control.

Kristi: I totally agree. The kids won't eat what we won't buy for them. Usually they don't know about flavored apples and blue yogurt. I'd say stick with the "Food Food" category. Buy apples that taste like apples check out plain yogurt and add blueberries a little honey.

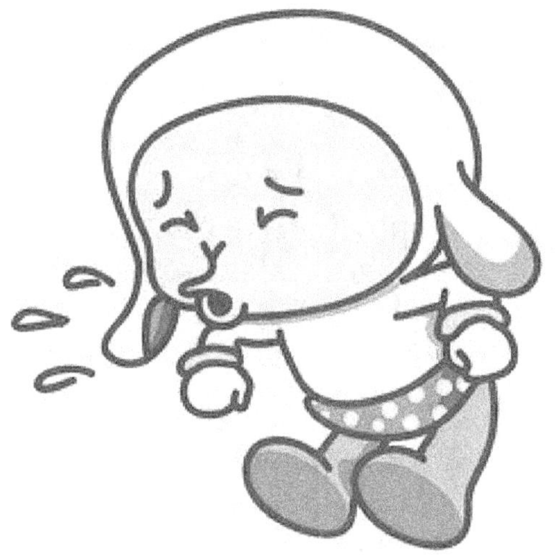

It's no wonder our kids are exploding with all kinds of crazy allergies and asthma; their little bodies aren't able to deal with all the chemicals. Ear infections, sinus infections, food allergies out of control. Inhalers and giving babies drugs with a syringe because they have reflux.

Maybe we should take notes from the kids, if it makes them throw up, we shouldn't eat it either!

Kristi: Now this next one hits at the very core of my old Americana, little pea pickin heart. We all grew up eating these little gems. Melt it on anything and you could get a kid to eat it. Even broccoli and cauliflower was able to be choked down by many a child once it was smothered in these.

Miriam: We never had this in Cuba we used Swiss cheese, but when we moved to the United States in the sixties I remember being so mesmerized by Velveeta. I had never seen anything like that, or canned ham for that matter.

Kristi: Oh yes. I was a big Velveeta eater. Of course, because we grew up with it never dawned on me what an odd thing that Velveeta "cheese" was stored on a shelf and not in the refrigerator.

I remember in college the first time going to the store to buy Velveeta and asking the clerk in the refrigerated area where the Velveeta was and he took me to the regular store shelf. I said, "It doesn't have to be refrigerated?" He said, "No, it's not really cheese."

Now check these little gems, Kraft Singles, this is a huge favorite of kids and adults everywhere. Who didn't grow up on grilled cheese? If we were going to get fancy we used the singles or Velveeta.

Kraft has a new campaign trying to appear natural and "Artisan", the new keyword for the big corporations trying to squeeze themselves into the "local artisan" grass roots movement. Kind of like a 7 foot tall basketball player trying to squeeze into a size 5 pair of red high heels.

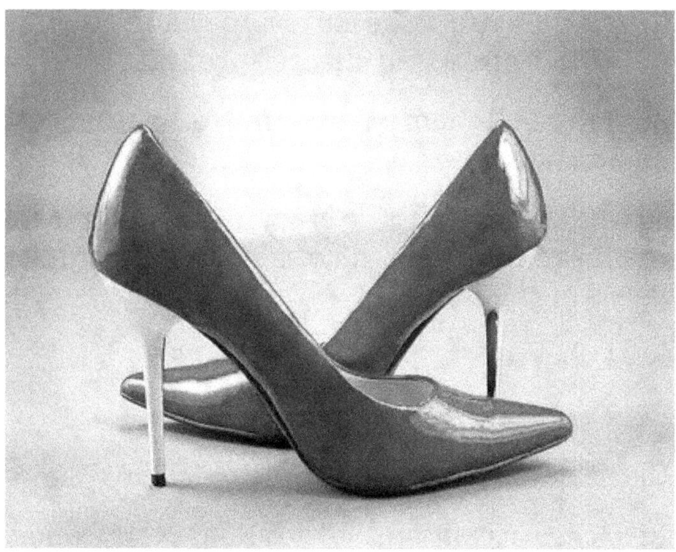

Yeah! We think it's pretty silly too.

Kraft says they took out artificial preservatives and use only natural preservatives, in the form of a "proprietary blend." Usually this means a chemical they patented, that comes from something natural in the beginning but have processed it so much it is now a chemical.

Kraft singles does have some milk in them but they have such a small amount of food in them, because it's mostly chemicals and milk by products, the FDA won't allow them to call it food...

That's why Kraft Cheese had to change their name to a processed cheese "product."

Miriam: Tell them what your Brother told you about cheese.

Kristi: Oh yes that's so crazy. My Brother is in the meat industry and he said there are three levels of cheese.

Real Cheese

Cheese Food

Cheese Product

Real cheese contains dairy, and is really food. The Cheese Food has added chemicals and preservatives.

The Cheese Product doesn't meet the Government's standards, not having enough food ingredients in it to even be called food.

Should your cheese read, "More Lab than Farm. No cow was involved in the making of this cheese."

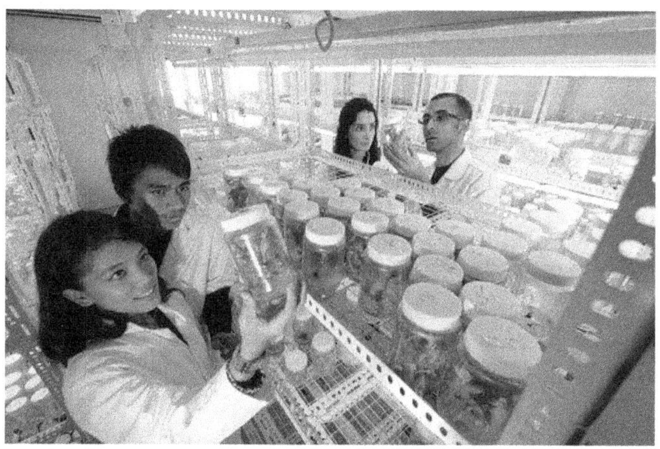

Kraft Singles Ingredients: Are in our "No Food" Category

Lots of No Food In here.

whey, milk, milk protein concentrate, milk fat, whey protein concentrate, sodium citrate, less than 2% of calcium phosphate, salt, lactic acid, annatto and paprika extract (color), natamycin, enzymes, cheese culture, and vitamin D3.

Is this in your fridge?

Miriam: Most people we have talked to that use Kraft singles do it out of convenience, grab it throw it in the cart unwrap it put it on some bread and they are ready to go. They feel like it saves time and money. It may save a fraction of a second but it definitely does not save money.

It's much cheaper to go to the deli ask them to slice some cheese, while they are slicing, do the rest of your shopping. Now you save time and you are paying for food not chemicals.

Miriam: It's amazing how many slices of cheese you get when you use the deli and you know that it hasn't been sitting on a storage shelf in some back room for a year.

Cheesy Little Shopping Tip

Cheddar is actually supposed to be white as is all cheese, it is made from cream and milk after all. When they turn it orange it is a coloring. It may not be harmful but if you don't need the orange color why have it? Also always buy full fat, the low fat kind not only tastes a bit wonky but they have to add chemicals to replace the fat.

A truly delectable cheese is Organic Valley Raw Sharp Cheddar Cheese in the block. If they don't have it at the deli to slice for you, grab a block in the organic section. We avoid pre shredded as well as there is usually cellulose (sometimes made from wood pulp) in there for an anti-caking agent.

Miriam: Remember that customer that would come into the restaurant and always brought his no fat cheese slices with him so we could put that on his food? His Doctor had him on all these no fat low fat food "items." They would buy bottled water and add these powder packets of flavorings to the water, the packets were also full of chemicals.

Kristi: It was so sad he couldn't eat salads because of his medicine and was eating all these "foods" that were nothing but chemicals. I don't know how we have all been convinced that fresh foods are not nearly as good for us as chemicalized "no foods."

Miriam: Slowly. We have been slowly fed a mental diet of giving ourselves over to the manufacturers and the doctors.

Doctors are wonderful and very necessary, but we must take responsibility for ourselves as well.

Less Truly is More.

Kristi: Yes. The key here is that you want to buy food with fat and calories and that will also rot. You want your cheese to mold that means that food which does go bad hasn't been saturated with so much "No Food" chemicals it can sit around till Jesus comes!

The less processing the more food.

We have students ask why it is that healthy food is so much more expensive than unhealthy food.

In reality it's not more expensive.

The unhealthy "food" is so full of chemicals that you aren't actually buying food.

There's No Food in Your Food!

You can buy cheese for a 1.00 a pack if you want plastic wrapped chemicals.

Don't believe us? Go to YouTube, put in the search "Kraft singles don't melt" and watch all the videos of people trying to melt them.

It's a video on Youtube of man trying to light a piece of cheese with a lighter. It was the processed cheese from a plastic wrap and they couldn't get the cheese to melt. It just burned and sizzled and looked more like plastic than something you should eat.

Recap:

The "Disease" you were diagnosed with may just be last night's dinner, and the night before and the night before. Your dinner doesn't have to be big, to give you a heart attack. Maybe it's the chemicals and processed salt.

If the Government makes a food manufacturer take the word FOOD off their item.

 Don't eat it.

Adults peeing on themselves is not something to be celebrated. And it is not inevitable.

Advertisers want to sell you a pill to "cure" your "disease." (Notice how much of the commercial talks about the dangerous side effects way longer than they talk about curing the "disease." Seems there's a New disease every week.)

Your body will not burn itself into destruction, you must stop running through the bushes dragging a torch (or twinkie) behind you setting the fires. Give your body a chance before you decide there is no hope for change.

After all if I can lose the weight I struggled with my entire life and get off blood pressure medicine, ANYTHING is possible!

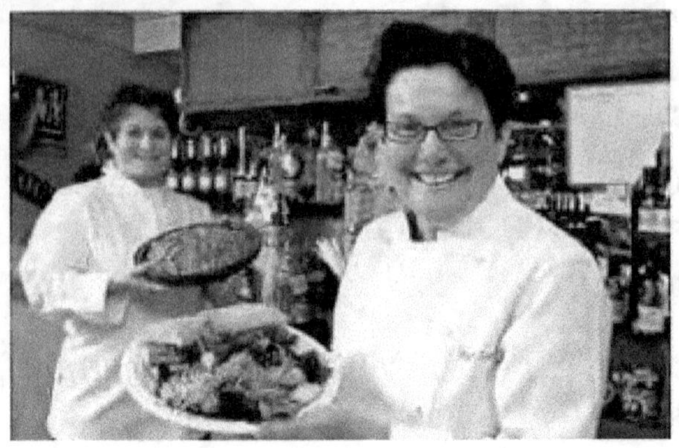

This is a great picture from the "old days" at our restaurant; this was from a Magazine interview about Miriam and her "Living the American Dream." They were featuring our café and her creation of Canary Island Garlic Herb Olive Oils.

That's me in the back I would say I was probably 220lbs in this picture, I later went on to "blossom" up to 240lbs.

How do you like that?

"Blossom" the first time I heard that "polite assessment of a woman's weight," was in church from a petite delicate-ish Grandmotherly type in the pew in front of me, when she leaned over and whispered to her friend, "My, my, my, hasn't she blossomed since last summer."

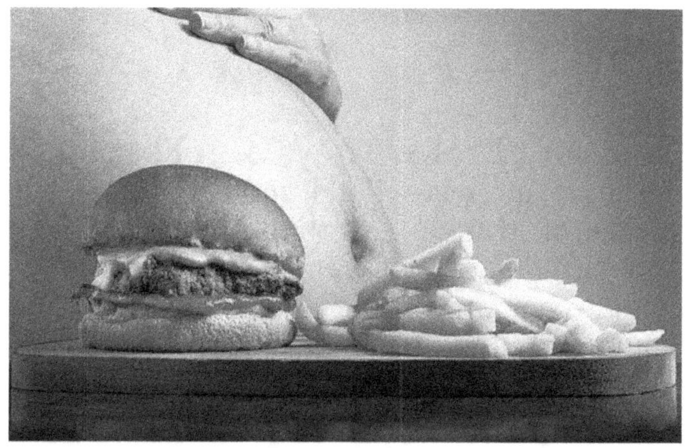

Kristi: Okay, so truth be told that is not a picture of me but when I saw this picture it so accurately portrayed part of how I got up to 240 lbs that I had to include it!

Miriam: It also looks exactly like it feels a lot of times when we speak to our students they tell us they feel like they are going to blow up, after they eat out.

Kristi: The craziest thing is you start to get use to feeling like that, because use to be I didn't think I was full until I couldn't breath!

Then I knew I was done eating. It's crazy now that I look back.

That is, afterall, the definition of crazy: "Doing the same thing over and over again and expecting different results."

Chapter 3

You Ain't Broke, They Can't Fix You

In this chapter we will tell some personal stories of struggle with all too common illnesses the diagnosis and how after a few simple changes, the "dis-ease ailments" completely disappeared.

Kristi: I hope you aren't getting tired of my stories, I always say if you survive, it will make a great story later!

True story. After all, you can't make this kind of crazy up! I went home to visit my Mom, since Miriam and I owned a restaurant the first thing out of my Mom's mouth, "I don't want you to think you are going be cooking while you're here. You are here to relax and enjoy your vacation. (Usually I like to cook up a bunch of goodies for her to freeze so she can nibble on them after I go home).

This time I gave in and didn't cook for a week. We ate out every meal except breakfast. We would do Mexican, Italian, good old American hamburgers, Pizza, couple of frozen dinners and some southern fried chicken. We were having fun and enjoying all the food until, I woke up one morning feeling not too well. To say the least.

I had noticed my joints were swollen, "Sausage Fingers" was back, I had to take my rings off every night, and my fingers had been swelling up over my rings. My ankles were swollen, I would take my sandals off it looked like I still had them on, my feet were so swollen. My back started hurting my knees felt tight and then the kicker.

Eating out sent me to the E.R

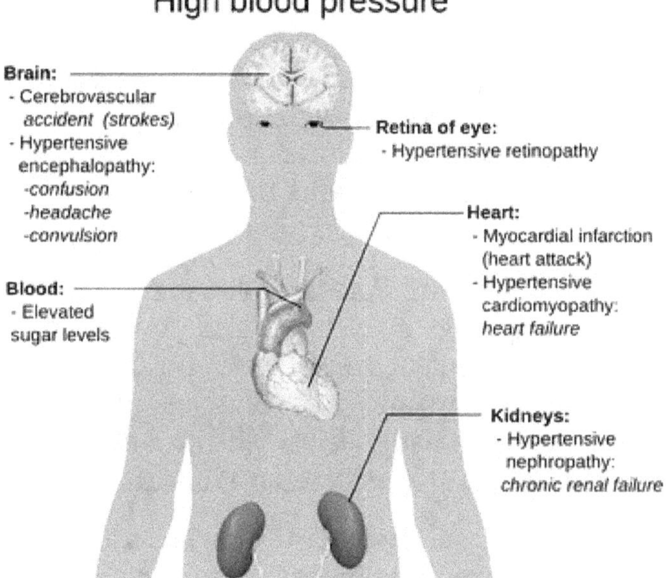

I woke up from my nap my heart rate was 100 and I had been sound asleep. I felt woozy my heart was skipping beats. It continued to get worse throughout the morning my Mom finally talked me into going to the Doctor. I ended up in the E.R.

I filled out the paperwork and from all my symptoms they thought I was having a heart attack. I mean, come on now I had just turned 40 but, this seemed just crazy.

To make a long story short I was put on blood pressure medicine and sent to a cardiologist. Meanwhile I spoke with Miriam.

Kristi: You tell them what you said.

Miriam: The first thing out of my mouth. Have you girls been eating out a lot? Because if you have, your condition has been chemically induced by food that contains artificial chemicals and ingredients to make it taste good but sure can kill you in the meantime.

It's not so much the food you eat it's what these companies do to make and preserve the food before you eat it. MSG and sodium are flavor enhancers and preservatives, plus hormones; the list goes on. The best choice is not to eat out and just prepare food at home.

You can juice celery and take garlic to lower your blood pressure. Now I'm no doctor but that's what I would did. And whatever you do, don't eat out. Fix meals with the Splash

(Canary Island Garlic and Herb Olive Oil Splash).

Canary Island Garlic and Herb Olive Oil contains only 15 mg of Sodium per serving. 10mg is classified Salt FREE!

Kristi: So the next day I started cooking all our meals with the Splash and drinking celery juice. Within a week my blood pressure had returned to normal.

 It was a very scary and extremely expensive lesson. They did a CT scan. At one point they wheeled me into a room and gave me some type of shot to lower my blood pressure. They said that if my pressure continued to rise and the bottom number reached the top number, I could have a stroke. Super Scary.

WARNING: Did you know that there are many "Low Sodium" foods that now use Potassium Chloride to lower the sodium count?

What's the big deal with Potassium Chloride?

The problem with it is that Potassium Chloride is used to lower blood pressure. So someone who is on blood pressure lowering medication should not be using Potassium Chloride. And no one should supplement with Potassium Chloride except under the care of a physician. Potassium is also very hard on your kidneys so if you suffer with diabetes and high blood pressure you absolutely should stay away from Potassium Chloride.

Kristi: Well check out this next item. I use to eat grilled cheese and tomato soup all the dern time. They were born to be eaten together. double whammy!

Miriam: NO food in your food for sure.

Campbell's Classic Healthy Request Tomato

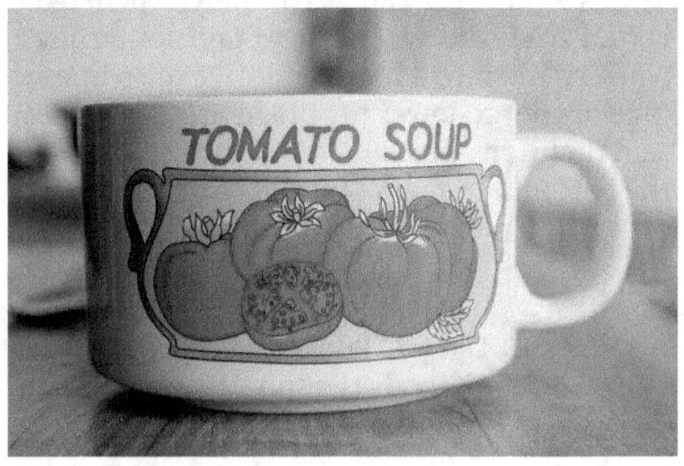

Lots of No Food in here.

TOMATO PUREE (WATER, TOMATO PASTE), WATER, WHEAT FLOUR, HIGH FRUCTOSE CORN SYRUP, CONTAINS LESS THAN 2% OF: SALT, POTASSIUM CHLORIDE, VEGETABLE OIL (CORN, COTTONSEED, CANOLA, AND/OR SOYBEAN), LOWER SODIUM NATURAL SEA SALT, FLAVORING, ASCORBIC ACID (VITAMIN

C), CITRIC ACID, MONOPOTASSIUM PHOSPHATE.

Did you see the Potassium Chloride in there? It is the 6th Ingredient, right after salt. Did you notice that salt is in there more than once. Check out the cottonseed oil.

Cottonseed oil is a manufacturing by-product from the cotton industry, it's *clearly not food.* And it's also linked to inflammation, which is linked to many known diseases.

We won't bore you with tons of label examples. But before you think it's just a soup problem. Read the next product. This one is for babies. If this doesn't put a streak of anger in your heart, then nothing will.

Our Children are our most precious gift

Lots of children grew up on formula and everybody thought they were giving their children something healthy to help them get a head start in life. It really has been touted as the way for our children to get all the best nutrients.

Somehow we have been convinced that a powdered substance that you can add water to and feed your baby is better than breast milk.

I know it will blow your mind when you read the chemicals in the baby formula. I'm not saying everybody has to breastfeed their children. I'm just saying, think about it and read the label before you make that decision.

Similac Unflavored Baby Formula

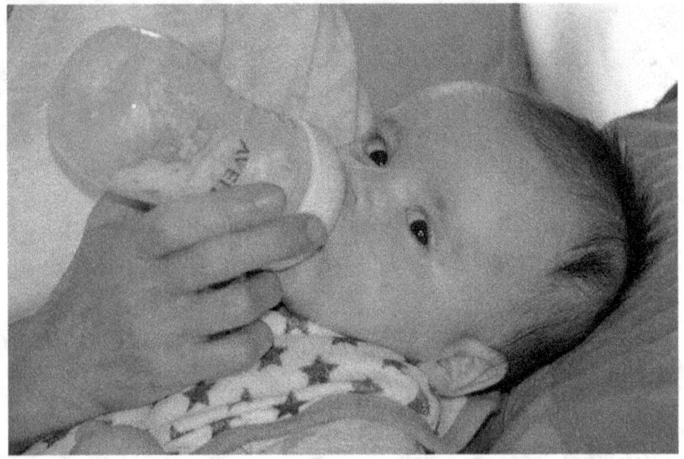

A Ton of No Food in here, maybe that's why they have to call it Baby "Formula" and not Food!

Nonfat Milk, Lactose, Whey Protein Concentrate, High Oleic Safflower Oil, Soy Oil, Coconut Oil, Galactooligosaccharides. Less than 2% of the Following: C. Cohnii Oil, M. Alpina Oil, Beta-Carotene, Lutein, Lycopene, Potassium Citrate, Calcium Carbonate, Ascorbic Acid, Soy Lecithin, Potassium Chloride, Magnesium Chloride, Ferrous Sulfate, Choline Bitartrate, Choline Chloride,

Ascorbyl Palmitate, Salt, Taurine, m-Inositol, Zinc Sulfate, Mixed Tocopherols, d-Alpha-Tocopheryl Acetate, Niacinamide, Calcium Pantothenate, L-Carnitine, Vitamin A Palmitate, Cupric Sulfate, Thiamine Chloride Hydrochloride, Riboflavin, Pyridoxine Hydrochloride, Folic Acid, Manganese Sulfate, Phylloquinone, Biotin, Sodium Selenate, Vitamin D3, Cyanocobalamin, Calcium Phosphate, Potassium Phosphate, Potassium Hydroxide, and Nucleotides (Adenosine 5'-Monophosphate, Cytidine 5'-Monophosphate, Disodium Guanosine 5'-Monophosphate, Disodium Uridine 5'-Monophosphate).

Did you see the Potassium Chloride? How about the cheapest oil, Soybean Oil is the 5th ingredient. We really need a chemist degree to read the label of the "formula" we are feeding them.

We could go on and on listing all the frozen dinners, salad dressings, cereals, boxed dinners and other baby formulas that contain not only Potassium Chloride but a toxic barrel of other chemicals. But, you get the point.

Consumption of Potassium Chloride has been found to cause heart palpitations and arrhythmia. Also has shown to result in confusion, anxiety, feeling like you might pass out, uneven heartbeat, extreme thirst, increased urination and leg discomfort.

Kristi: Wow I wasn't expecting all that in a can of soup! Or a baby bottle.

I remember when Miriam started noticing all these products listing high potassium. She started researching it through restaurant and other industry journals, she found the reason.

 All these big manufacturers were promoting the use of Potassium Chloride instead of Sodium Chloride so they could list the sodium as being lower. Pretty scary!

Miriam: It is crazy. I kept noticing the potassium counts. I'm so glad we figured it out and can share it with our students.

When you start reading the ingredients you will almost always find potassium chloride and salt and sea salt and other forms, sodium bicarbonate etc.

All in the same product! What people don't realize is these are drugs that pharmaceutical companies make, that are being put in the food.

Don't take any medications?

 You think you don't take any medications, but if you eat processed foods you are loading up on a medicine chest full of drugs.

That's not even mentioning all the interactions that these drugs have with drugs you do take. The potassium chloride found in many foods reacts with other drugs enhancing effects of the other drugs.

417 known medications interact with Potassium Chloride.

2806 brand name and generic drugs interact with Potassium Chloride.

You can go to www.drugs.com and enter a medication to see if it interacts in a mild to severe way.

"Potassium Chloride is the drug used in Lethal Injection, to stop the heart."

Kristi: It is mind boggling that a lot of side effects of these drugs they put in food are symptoms of major diseases. Like frequent urination and thirst. Then there is heart palpitations, arrhythmia, dizziness and confusion to name a few.

Miriam: Sounds a lot like many disease symptoms like AFib for one, some of those symptoms can be dizziness, fatigue fast heart rate or sensation of abnormal heartbeat, weakness and shortness of breath.

Kristi: That is crazy. You could actually be diagnosed with a disease and be given a drug regimen and maybe it is what you are eating. That is insane isn't it?

Miriam: I have seen many of my peers fall between the cracks and end up with a grocery bag of medications.

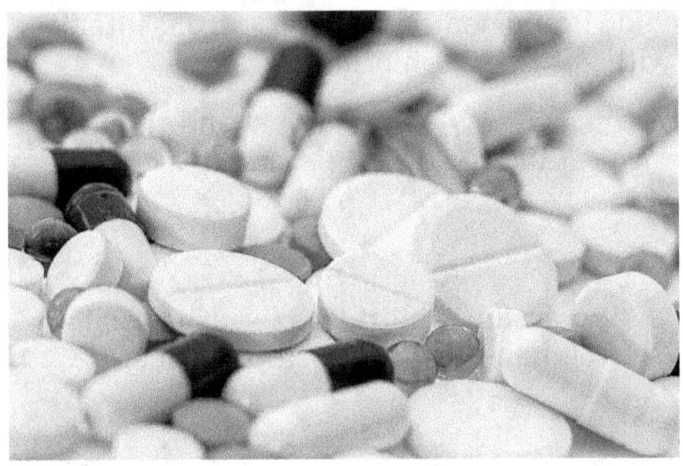

Back to our story:

Needless to say, the next two weeks I was on vacation we ate at home every day. I am relieved to tell you I am no longer on blood pressure medicine and the swelling achy joints went away as well.

One of the shots they gave me was an anti-anxiety drug to relax me to lower my blood pressure. They sent me home with anti-anxiety pills.

I had no idea what was going on. The shot really relaxed me and the pills kept me floating around. I didn't like the weird feeling it gave me.

Kristi: I have struggled with anxiety most of my life everybody always called be a scaredy cat!

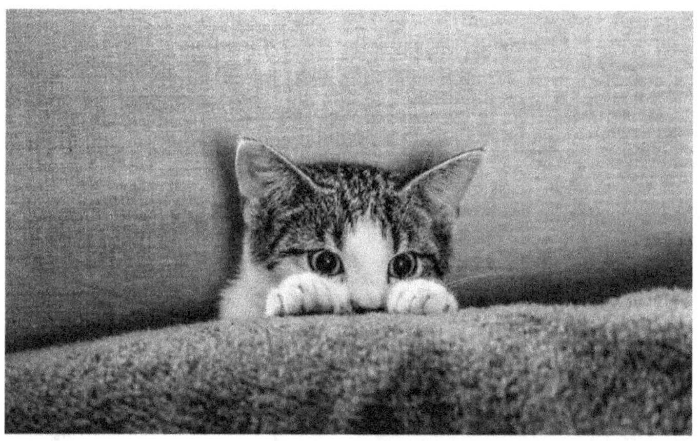

 I can all too well relate to people who struggle with daily anxiety and anxiety attacks.

I remember one incident in college during class I had an anxiety attack hit me so hard, I had to have a friend hold my hand and take me to the bathroom and stay with me until I could breathe again.

I am so grateful to her. It's kind of humorous now that I think of it. We were both getting our Social Work Degrees and she sat in that bathroom talking me through the attack.

Miriam: I guess you could say that you got on the job training. Thank Goodness she was there to help you.

Kristi: Exactly.

Here is an example. Have you ever experienced this?

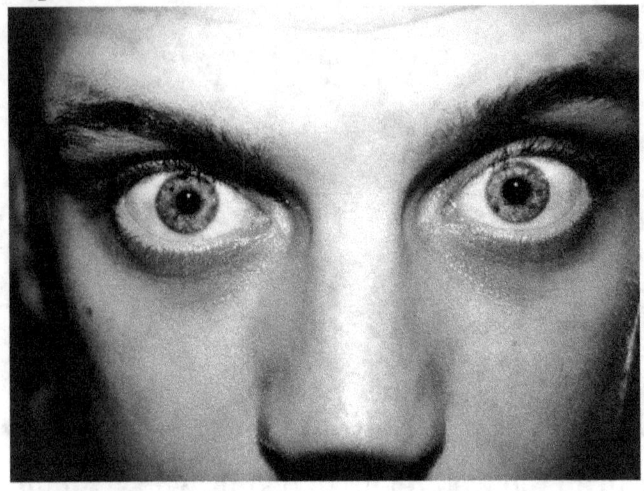

 Your heart suddenly starts pounding the cold sweat rolling down your sides, your brain starts a cyclone of dark thoughts that don't shut off. Then every ache every noise every bad thought that could possibly ever happen in a million years, becomes real.

Suddenly the remark somebody made at work is blown out of proportion and your brain rolls around in the deep with that thought like an

Anaconda taking down its prey. Then your kids quick answer turns into a smart remark and your spouses inquisitive look becomes an accusing eye. Everything happening around you becomes a personal attack.

I know that's how it was for me.

Kristi: I am thankful that over the years when I did use anxiety medication, I never became addicted. Addiction, unfortunately is all too often the end result.

Xanax and its siblings—Valium, Ativan, Klonopin... family of drugs called benzodiazepines—suppress the output of neurotransmitters that interpret fear.

They differ... in potency and duration; those that enter your brain most quickly (Valium and Xanax) can make you the most high.

But all quell the racing heart, spinning thoughts, prickly scalp, and hyperventilation associated with fear's neurotic cousin, anxiety, and all do it more or less instantly.

Prescriptions ... have risen to... 94 million a year; generic Xanax, called alprazolam, has increased... making it the most prescribed psycho-pharmaceutical drug..., with 46 million prescriptions written in 2010.

In their generic forms, *Xanax* is prescribed more than the sleeping pill Ambien, more than the antidepressant Zoloft. Only drugs for chronic conditions like high blood pressure and high

cholesterol do better (are prescribed more).
<u>Nymag.com</u>

It's truly amazing when I stopped eating so
many chemicals my anxiety totally and
completely vanished. Faster than a teenager,
asked to do the dishes!

Miriam: I tell our students all the time. "You
Are Not Broken." Don't allow yourself to fall
through the cracks. Either you take control of
your diet and what you put into your mouth.
Or, later on, you will give control to the
Doctors and you will have to pay them to dig
all the bad stuff out.

Kristi: I am still amazed that I lost all that
weight and have kept it off for over 2 years.
Taking the chemicals out and a few other little
tweeks you showed me has completely
changed my life. Not only have I "fixed"
myself by getting rid of all those "Dinner
Time Diseases." But I lost 35 lbs. over the
summer for a total of 70lbs.

No Exercise. No Sweat. No Drama. No Fasting.
No Shakes. No Work.

Kristi: What an Absolutely Fantastic "Side
Effect!"

Recap:

Anxiety is not forever. Fat is Not Forever. But you can be Forever Free of Fat and Anxiety.

More No Food than food= dinnertime disease.

Just because everyone eats it doesn't mean they feel good.

Eating chemicals that are used in Lethal Injection is Not a good idea... Ever

Kristi: Being free of anxiety is a gift greater than I can describe. If you have never suffered with anxiety it is hard to relate a terror of such magnitude and feeling of impending doom and destruction from, an unseeable force. If you have suffered with anxiety or still do, there is Hope, it doesn't have to be that way. I now live on the other side of that dark night.

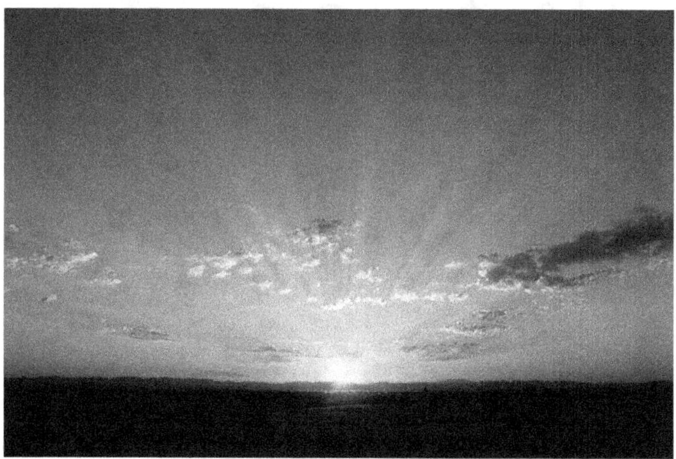

Chapter 4

There is No Food in Your Food

In this chapter we bust wide open the "No Food" theory. When you buy a bowl of "Food" from a restaurant or pre-packaged you are really buying a crock full of...something else. Bam Boom Pow!

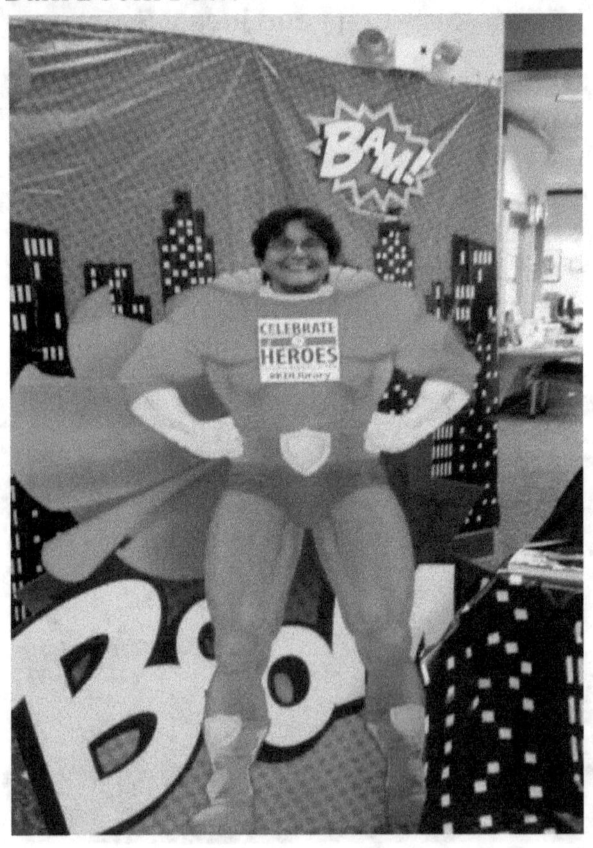

As a child my family's menu consisted of 2 choices: take it or leave it. ~ Buddy Hackett

It's not like the old days, when your Mom or Dad cooked dinner breakfast and lunch. What they made was what you ate. They would normally make a meat lots of fresh veggies from the garden and homemade bread.

It's easy to get sucked into the black hole of no time to cook; we all have 300 things on our to-do list. We have kids, cats or dogs, errands, and the extra mile at work. Many Americans have two jobs, so add that to the pile.

 It's so much easier to run through the drive thru, grab a frozen dinner and pop in the micro. If the food available at the drive thru and the frozen food department was just food, it wouldn't be so bad.

Unfortunately for us, most of the food in the drive thru and frozen food department are made up of more chemicals and preservatives than actual digestible food.

Remember:

More Chemicals, more processed oils, more sugar, more salt= More Inflammation

More Inflammation=More Disease

More Disease=More Pain

FYI:

McDonald's Oatmeal lists 21 ingredients, four of which are barley malt extract and caramel color, maltodextrin and carrageenan (otherwise known as MSG). MSG is a concentrated form of salt often linked to allergic reactions. MSG is 12.2% sodium.

Kristi: We have spoken to so many people, when we ask them if they eat MSG they say. "I don't eat Chinese food." So they think they aren't getting MSG. The truth is if you eat boxed, manufactured, processed food and always if you eat out. You are ABSOLUTELY eating MSG!

Miriam: People wonder why they can't breathe when they finish eating at a restaurant. They have heart palpitations get nauseated or have diarrhea. That's MSG.

So imagine, products that list MSG under different names and all the times salt is listed by different names. So, there really is no food in your food.

TIP OF THE DAY:

Instead of grabbing a package of instant oatmeal with weird apple cinnamon flavoring or grabbing it at the fast food chain, which will usually end up being ordered with a hash brown and sausage biscuit.

Do This:

Boil water. Put old fashioned oatmeal in. Stir.
Turn off heat. Put lid on. Let steam while you
finish getting dressed.

Put Canary Island Garlic Herb Olive Oil in a
pan and pop an egg on top till cooked. Serve
on top of oatmeal.

Or, overnight oats with berries. What a great
way to start your day, full of "Food Food!"

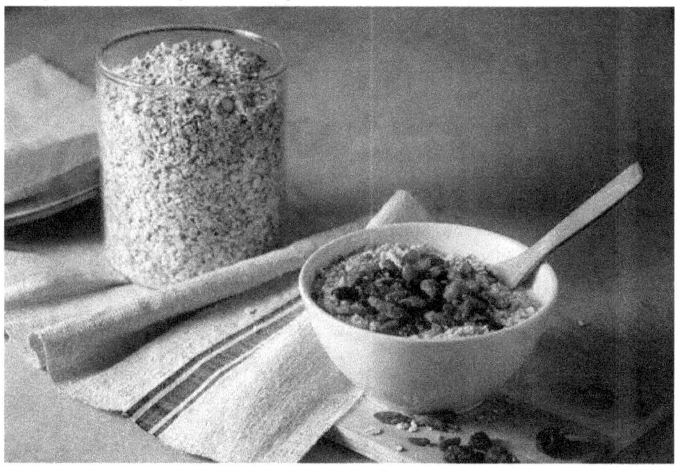

FYI

McDonald's ended up getting sued by State
Officials in Vermont for stating that they were
using Maple in their Maple oatmeal, even
though they never put any Maple in there.

Kristi: Holy Chemical Stew, Batman! That is Crazy, 21 ingredients for a little bowl of, "McDonald's Healthy" oatmeal. I think I will just stick to my old fashioned oatmeal cooked in water and sprinkled with cinnamon or Canary Island Olive Oil.

Miriam: You know, when you say old fashioned, that is exactly how these manufacturers want you to feel. The cozy feeling of sitting around Grandma's table her homemade cooking and all the warm fuzzies related to the old fashioned meal.

The homemade macaroni and cheese, the homemade peach cobbler, the homemade bread and sliced turkey sandwich from leftover Thanksgiving dinner.

If you notice, the "Old Fashioned" comfort foods are packed on the grocery store convenience aisles. But now days the comfort foods will give you discomfort later when your blood pressure shoots through the roof.

The manufacturers are playing on your memories and longings to have the "Good Old Days" again.

But they process the "food" so much then add chemicals and fake flavors and tons of salt to make it super cheap and still taste like something. Here's the problem with there being "No Food in Your Food," and nothing but chemicals...

You are ALWAYS hungry!

Kristi: I don't know about you but after I ate out or had cereal for breakfast or maybe a McGriddle from McDonalds. I Could Eat the Curtains off the Wall, after I had finished eating the tablecloth.

So you eat and eat and eat and your kids are whiny and hungry you grab a Nugget at your local McD's and you feed them and they need more because they are starving for nutrition but are ending up with chemicals that make them crave more food!

Speaking of our children, Macaroni and Cheese, Food Babe just wrote a blog post of the 22 different ingredients found in Easy Mac and Cheese by Kraft. Crazy list of MSG and GMOs and other crazy preservatives and chemicals are packed into the food marketed specifically for kids. Like Food Babe says, as far as we knew mac and cheese was butter, milk, cheese and noodles!

Kristi: Oh and let's not forget that's the one they want you to pop in the microwave for the kids!

 Let's grab an orange juice for the kids, that's healthy right? I was reading an article the other day about the orange juice makers.

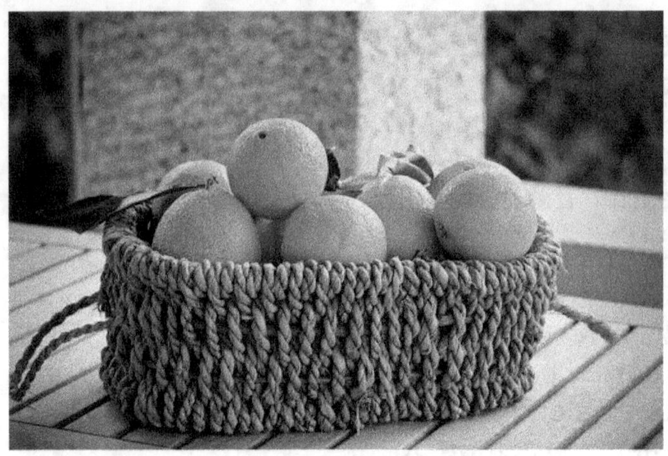

We all remember home squeezed orange juice growing up. Now the OJ in the stores is about as fresh as a petrified toad. They store the "OJ" in large vats for up to one year.

True story.

Did you know? Orange juice you buy in the stores has been so overly processed they actually have to hire "perfume" makers to come in and make a chemical that makes the orange juice smell like orange juice should smell. Then they add it to the orange juice storage vat.

The reason they don't have to list the perfume as an ingredient on the label is because it is chemically related to the orange juice.

Miriam: Well that just stinks. The only thing you are drinking in your morning orange juice is a perfumed glass of sugar. That's a sour pill to swallow.

Back to the MSG in the McDonald's oatmeal. The MSG is used for everything from coloring to texture, fillers to preservatives in many foods, not just their oatmeal. I also recently found out that salt is processed in different ways so they can use it to color or to give texture or bulk as well.

MSG is made by a series of chemical reactions using genetically engineered bacteria.

"Its new oatmeal, which McDonald's released nationwide last month as a "bowl full of wholesome," is actually a crock full of something else, according to Mark Bittman, author of the new book, "Vegan B46", and blogger for The New York Times."

"It's put forward as this wholesome thing when, in fact, it's sort of an amalgam of ingredients you wouldn't ordinarily have at home," he said.

The oatmeal bought in any grocery store across the country only has one ingredient, oats

 But McDonald's oatmeal has 21 ingredients, including natural flavor, barley malt extract and caramel color.

"I think it's misleading to portray this as a healthy breakfast because the McDonald's oatmeal has about the same amount of sugar as a Snickers bar, has about the same amount of calories as one of their hamburgers, costs more than one of their hamburgers," Bittman said. "It's just an odd way to go about serving a healthy breakfast."

Let's skip down to Treat Time:

Kristi: Funny Story. Before we look at the Wendy's ingredient list I have to tell you a story.

 When I was 13 years old my neighbor Lisa and I would ride our bikes up to Wendy's and get Frosties. That was our favorite bike ride. It was kind of a long ride and all up hill, of course.

Miriam: Was it uphill both ways? Ha Ha.

Kristi: No ha ha. But the great thing about that ride it was really hot and it was always great to have a really hot hard ride and then go in and order our Frosties and then ride downhill all the way home and eat them while swinging in the shaded backyard in our hammock.

This particular Frosty foray we were almost all the way back to my house and about a block away. The bottom of the paper bag that was holding my beloved Frosty, fell out and out toppled my Frosty. AAAh Salvation the lid stayed on and it didn't spill. Right as I'm rejoicing in the strength of the lid I ran over the Frosty with my back tire!

Miriam: Oh No! How funny.

Kristi: Funny! I was traumatized. Ha ha and Lisa didn't share her Frosty. My Mom made us watermelon slices to make up for the trauma.

Miriam: Well you were healthy that day anyway.

Kristi: True, True.

Peek inside: Wendy's Frosty 17 ingredients with MSG listed several times:

Milk, Cream, Sugar, Corn Syrup, Cocoa (processed with alkali), Guar Gum, Mono and Diglycerides, Cellulose Gum, Dextrose, Carrageenan, Calcium Sulfate, Disodium Phosphate, Artificial and Natural Flavor, Vitamin A Palmitate. CONTAINS: MILK.

Miriam: Solution: Make your own. I love this frozen coffee, we would make at our restaurant to rave reviews. I took mine with espresso for sure.

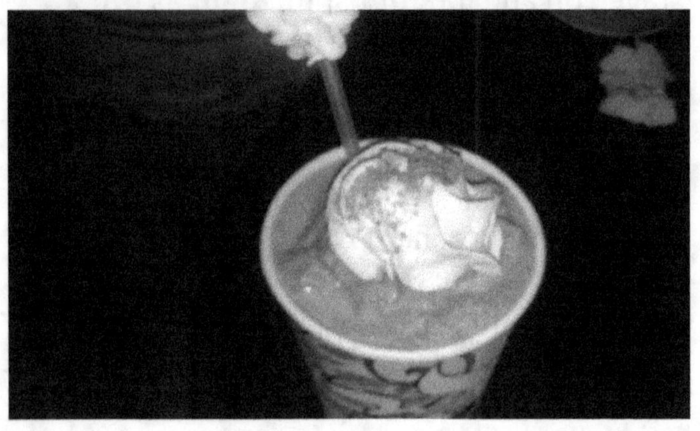

TIP OF THE DAY: Ditch the "NO FOOD" Frosty and make a Frozen Coffee of the Gods!

1 Cup Almond Milk

1 shot of Espresso or strong coffee (3oz)

2 shakes of cinnamon

2 Frozen Bananas

Blend until Fabulous.

If you don't like coffee leave it out. I like to sometimes throw a couple of squares of dark chocolate and peanut butter in! If you like it thicker, while the blender is running, add a bit of ice or more banana. If you like it a bit sweeter always be sure to add overripe bananas and drizzle of honey. I have also used a Medjool date or two, make sure they don't have a pit in them.

Aldi has really great Medjool dates, leave out the honey or maple if you use dates they are plenty big and plenty sweet all by themselves.

Want to healthy-fy it up a bit? Add a ½ small avocado to the blender it makes it creamy and the fat will help slow down the digestion.

It's the funniest thing.

Adding the half avocado isn't really even noticeable, if you have added chocolate it will make the drink a little darker but it makes it almost fluffy like a marshmallow drink.

Miriam: I like avocado in my smoothies also, I don't care for sweet smoothies so the avocado works really well in my guava and mango shakes.

Kristi: And if you throw in a bit of spinach well now your body will feel over the moon with energy and your waistline will think you as well.

Do you know what a salt lick is?

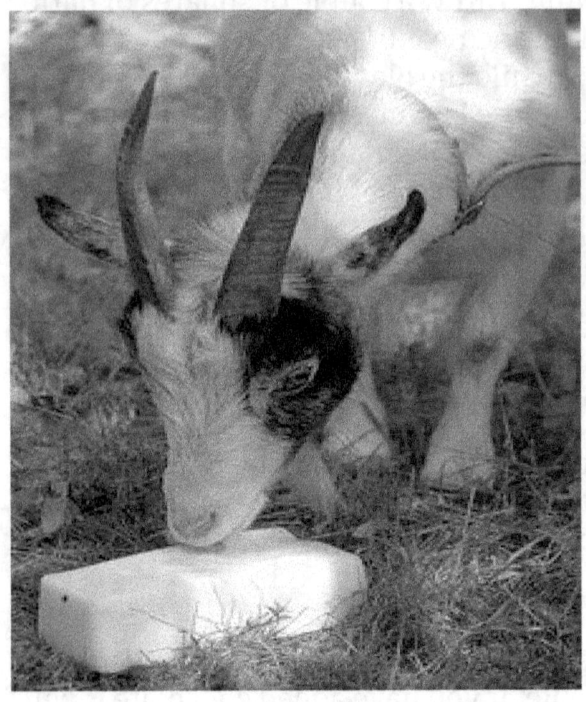

Definition of Salt Lick: noun. A block of salt provided for animals to lick.

Have you had one for dinner? Of course not.

Are you sure?

Kristi: I think I secretly had one snuck into my supper last night. We are writing this while we are on the road doing our cooking classes and seminars. We have to eat out when we are on location and we can't cook for ourselves. Even though I asked for no seasoning and no salt on the food. I woke up this morning with puffy eyes and cheeks.

Miriam: You look a lot like the little chipmunk that we have been feeding bananas to today.

Kristi: Yeah! No he looks cuter with puffy cheeks than I do. Does that ever happen to you?

Miriam: Well I get the puffy eyes, actually I also get dry eyes. A lot of people think they naturally have dry eyes and take prescription drops. I notice I get dry eyes when I'm eating out a lot and they are heavy on the msg and salt. Of course you don't know they are until the next morning!

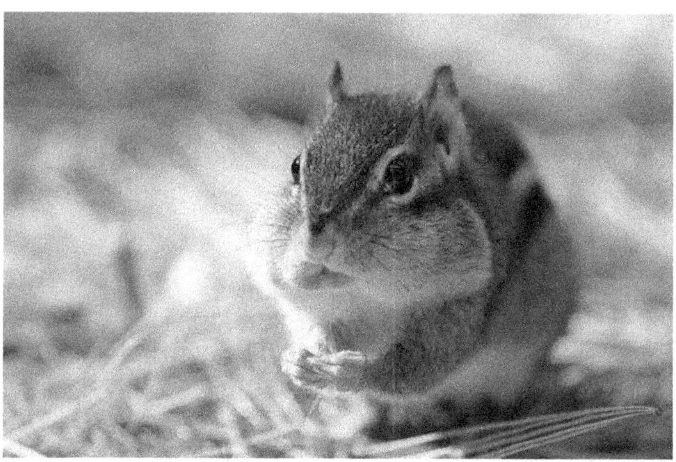

Kristi: You may find this hard to believe but I never realized how much salt that other restaurants put into their food.

Miriam and I owned a healthy restaurant for over 20 years, we ate there every day that we worked, and we both cook at home when we weren't at the restaurant. So the effects of the salt are very noticeable.

We do grab a slice of pizza or a hamburger every now and again, yes we usually feel bloated, swollen, gassy, and achy and my heart palpitates when we do it.

We are teaching chefs so we travel a lot, yes we have eaten at many a Cracker Barrel. We seem to do better at the Ruby Tuesday, you can load up on the salad section and get lots of fresh raw veggies.

Just remember to tell them no seasoning and no lemon butter, they season and drizzle lemon butter over everything before they serve. I'm not really sure if it's actual lemon and butter, so we avoid it.

Eating out Trick

Ask for a side of fresh lemons or limes and squeeze over your food for a bit of zest.

Kristi: Or you can do like a lot of our students and my Mom do, take a small amount of

Canary Island Garlic Herb Olive Oil with them and drizzle it over their food. Deelish!

Miriam: It's not that we are saying that you should never eat out or grab a convenient snack. It's to be aware of finding the snacks with the least amount of chemicals and fillers. Or if you find no other option, do as Kristi and I do and split the meal.

Kristi: At least at that point you are cutting everything in half.

Untouched by Human Hands ☺

Always try to order unprocessed food. Like a baked potato instead of mashed, usually mash is premade and has lots of "No Food" chemicals. Order sweet potato, instead of sweet potato fries.

Order a steak instead of a hamburger, or grilled trout without seasoning instead of fried fish or fish fillet.

Kristi: As far as I know, fish don't usually wear Panko crumbs in nature.

Miriam: Well maybe in Alaska when it's really cold! Ha ha

 If you order steamed veggies be aware that they are microwaving them in a premade seasoning in a plastic bag. Many times when we request no seasoning on the steamed veggies they will tell us that they seasoned them in the morning before they were put into the bags.

Most of the time the seasoning is a type of garlic or lemon butter composition, you can pretty much guarantee that it is not actual butter and lemon. If the steamed veggies are the healthiest choice then just go with the flow. Don't go with the bacon and potato stuffed soup instead.

Kristi: Ha Ha I have totally done that! Like you are on a diet and you make a little boo boo and instead of jumping back onto your good eating plan, I would say, "Well blew that one today I might as well eat a box of ice cream." Wait what?

TIP OF THE DAY:

Ask for no seasoning at all. If you need to tell them you are allergic, do it to make sure you are chemical free.

Kristi: I remember an interesting fact we discovered when we were on the road teaching and doing shows, we would occasionally eat at Subway.

I said to Miriam, "I don't feel good after I eat at all these restaurants let's just run into Subway."

So we grab a 6 inch Turkey sub with Provolone, who knew that a "healthy turkey" sandwich from Subway actually has 1,220mg of sodium, that's without the chips.

A bag of Doritos has 570 mg of sodium for one bag. Remember we are only talking about the sodium in the Doritos not all the crazy MSG and other chemicals.

After all a long list of chemicals is rather boring dinner conversation. ;-)

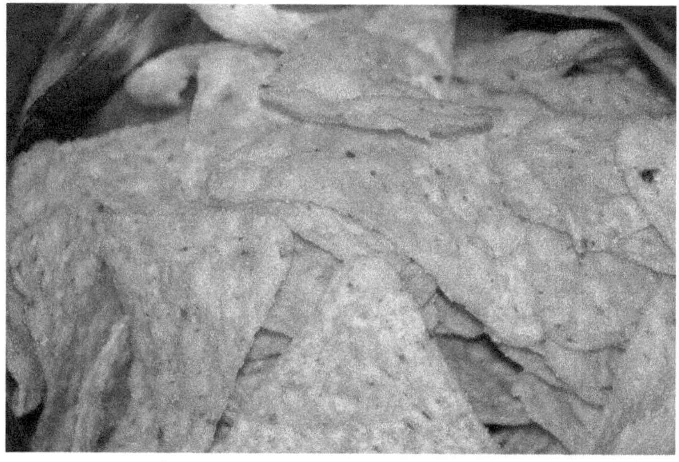

Of course you need a drink so you grab a diet coke and you added 40mg. So my quick "healthy" lunch at subway added up to 1,830mg of sodium.

We love food! I think we all have a special place in our hearts for a great meal and good conversation. We celebrate a win around the table, we grieve a loss around the table.

In times of hardship we bring hot food to warm the heavy heart. We take our very life nourishment from food. What's not to love?

Unfortunately, these facts will make your heart grow heavy.

Miriam: Did you know that the American Heart Association recommends no more than 2,300mg of sodium a day for healthy people and if you are over 50, African American or have kidney disease, high blood pressure or diabetes, you should have no more than 1,500mg a day. That's for the entire day.

Kristi: I would say play it safe and follow the stricter guidelines of 1,500mg. No matter who you are or what you have this way you are in the safe zone. When you have a splurge night you have a little wiggle room.

With one turkey sandwich from Subway I just ate up over half my days' worth of sodium, if I am playing it safe, I ate over my entire day's sodium. So after my Turkey sandwich lunch from Subway equaling 1,830mg of sodium I only have 470mg left that I can eat for the rest of the day.

Of course that is only if I don't grab the 3 for $1 Otis Spunkmeyer sugar cookies for later, for three cookies it will cost an additional 490 mg of sodium.

I just ate my entire days' worth of sodium in one meal at Subway and am already 20mg into tomorrow's sodium intake.

I bet you have Never said to yourself.

 I guess I better just have ice water the rest of the day!

Kristi: How in the world can a turkey sandwich have 1,830mg of sodium in one serving?

Regular turkey from the actual turkey, we call it Turkey Turkey has more protein and less fat than deli turkey.

A HUGE difference in Sodium. Turkey from the actual turkey.

"Turkey Turkey" has only 55 mg of sodium per 4 oz,

Deli turkey has 1,049mg of sodium!

Deli meat is so high in sodium because most of what you are eating in the deli meat is not actually meat but "No Food" chemicals! That's also why the protein is lower in deli meat than real turkey!

Kristi: Did you hear that? The protein in deli turkey is lower than the protein in Turkey Turkey. For gosh sakes!

You literally get less meat in Deli Turkey than you do in Turkey Turkey.

Miriam: You see this is a prime example that real food like Turkey Turkey will keep you full longer and you will eat less Food Food.

It's the "No Food" that keeps you hungry because chemicals will Never satisfy the soul of your stomach like good Food Food will.

Miriam: My Family has a saying, "It's cheaper to clothe you than to feed you!" So true, so true.

Manufacturers want to make as much money off of you and their turkey, cheese and bread as possible. The old fashioned way of cutting turkey off the bone for a sandwich was not profitable enough for the mega companies.

 So, they take the turkey mix it with chemicals, fillers, additives and preservatives (salt) sodium nitrate, grind, pulverize liquefy and remold the gelatinous mess into a "roast-like" shape and feed it to us. If you are eating sliced turkey you are eating all the turkey waste as well, tripe (intestines) brains and other ground turkey waste.

The fillers and additives give the turkey taste and help the pieces and parts glue together. Some of these reshaped turkey slices have 10% "juices added" or "solution added" which means salt water.

It is a cheap way to make 1 turkey feed a mob, but that shortcut is cutting our lives short.

You can pay $8.99 for one pound of this "fake No Food jiggly-meat" or buy an entire 12lb turkey for 11.99!

 That's 1.00/lb. for actual meat. "Turkey Turkey" for 1.00/lb.

Kristi: Now that is something to gobble about!

Miriam: Or you could pay $107.88 plus tax for 12 lb of "fake No Food meat".

Kristi: Well that ought to nauseate the budget conscious you!

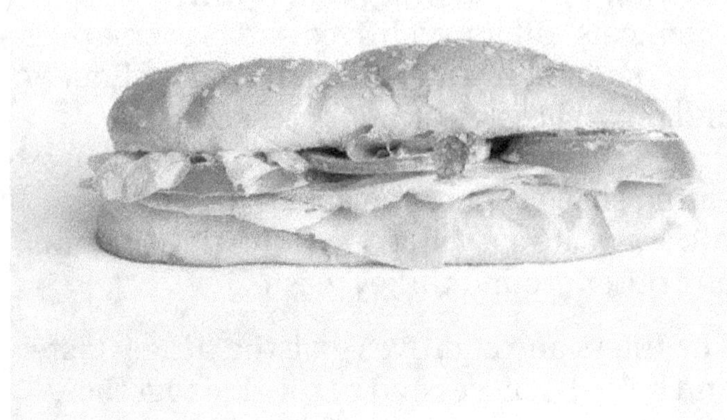

Peek inside: Tyson Chicken Rotisserie Deli Slices

25 Ingredients,

Chicken breast, chicken broth (water, powdered cooked chicken with natural flavor), vinegar, contains 2% or less of dextrose, salt, modified potato starch, corn syrup solids, carrageenan, sodium phosphates, onion and garlic powder, sodium erythorbate, brown sugar, chicken flavor (maltodextrin, salt, natural flavor), sodium nitrite, chicken fat, yeast extractive, glucose, spice extractive.)

Recap:

All processed meats are going to have salts and chemicals. Meat from the bone is best.

If it sits on a shelf in the grocery it probably sat somewhere else for a long time before it got there.

Old Fashioned Flavor is more old, than Flavor.

Home Style has been styled somewhere but not at Home, for sure.

Want fresh Orange Juice, get an Orange and Juice it. Apples? Carrots? You can juice those too. Or even better just eat the fruit, then you get the fiber as well.

Helpful Hint:

Once a month or every two weeks depending on your family size, cook a turkey breast or a whole turkey. Slice it up and freeze it. If you are off on Saturday or Sunday that's a great day or do it in the evening after work.

You can slice it or shred it, use it in your eggs your soups your wraps and your sandwiches. Use it cold on a sandwich or simply chop it up and add to your salad.

Be sure to get the unseasoned turkey.

Chapter 5

What is Making My Kid so Fat?

In this chapter we will reveal the reason why we "Just can't seem to help our kids lose the weight!"

Kristi: As the "Fat Kid". I know within the core of my being how miserable it is to be the "Fat Kid."

 It's not like wearing a shirt with a hole in it and being made fun of that day. It never goes away, you can't take off your Fat Shirt when you get home. The constant teasing and bullying I still remember, and I am 47 years old.

Miriam: It is such a heart break for parents whose children are overweight. They can't do anything to defend their children and can only try to console them when they are crumpled to tears. It is a relief to know that kids can follow these guidelines and lose the weight as easily as you did.

Kristi: I hope that all the parents who read this book will grab the possibility and really embrace the amazing change that is available for their kids, simply kick the "No Food" food to the curb. The results will be unbelievable.

Miriam: In a very short amount of time, your life was changed. You lost the 35lb in just 3 months wasn't it?

Kristi: Yes. And it continues to be the easiest thing I have ever done. We will have to share more about the simple style of eating you created.

Miriam: That is a great idea. You know I really want people to realize what these foods have in them and when they see them I want them to say," There is No Food in This Food. Should I Strip Paint With It Or Feed It To My Children?"

FYI: At one time there was a bill before Congress that attempted to expose the manufacturers that are pumping the meat products with salt water. At least if they are honest about pumping the meat with salt we as consumers can make an educated decision. So far no such regulations have come to pass.

Sliced Deli Meat Turkey No better than SPAM!

Spam: the butts of jokes, the gross gelatinous canned meat that we have all had as children and many people still have as adults.

Crazy Statistic

 3.8 cans of Spam are consumed every second in the United States.

Shocking to think, that many people still eat spam, with a sodium intake per serving of 1,368mg of sodium. People are eating 57% of their daily recommended dose of salt in just 3.5oz.

What's more shocking is that some sliced Turkey on average for 3.5oz to 4.0oz is around 1,400mg of sodium per serving.

Kristi: It's No wonder I was going to spin class working out at the gym and drinking a gallon of water we even hired a personal trainer and I was still busting at the seams. All those 4:00 a.m. workouts were not my most favorite way to start my day, for sure. We think we are being healthy ordering sliced turkey, when we are actually eating the equivalent of SPAM in disguise.   How Disgusting.

Here's the best use for a can of SPAM in my opinion.

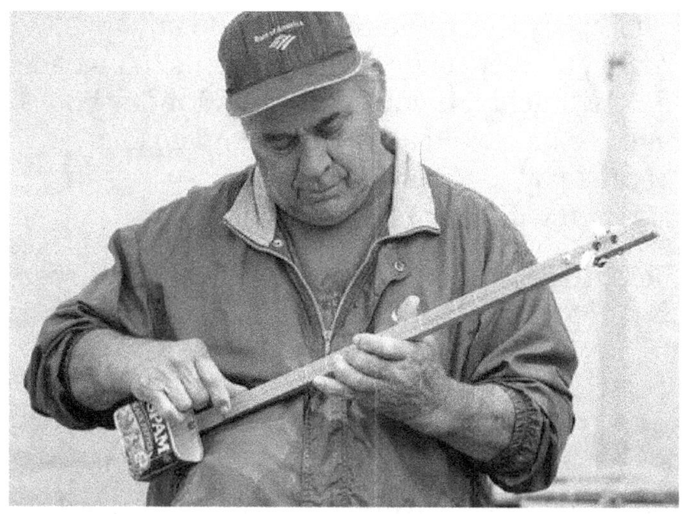

Miriam: I find it just crazy that people eat all this deli meat and feel like they are eating healthy. It's the sodium sneaking up on them.

Kristi: Like I always say, life is complicated enough, feeding yourself shouldn't be!

A surprise we found at the grocery store:

Years ago our customers started asking for turkey so we carried sliced turkey, we would buy it in bulk and slice it at the restaurant for our sandwiches and wraps.

Being in the food business we are very aware of shelf life: how many days you have to sell an item before it's considered bad.

The funny thing about turkey and any meat really, but especially turkey, seems to go bad pretty quickly. If you slice it on Monday you need to have sold all of it by late Tuesday because by Wednesday it's going to be slimy and you will have to pitch it.

Red meat is not bad for you. Now blue-green meat, now that's bad for you! ~ Tommy Smothers

Why is there such a short shelf life on sliced meat? It's because once you slice it and it is exposed to air it begins to deteriorate.

That being said, the turkey, ham or whatever lunch meat you eat, already has a lot of preservatives, nitrates and nitrites in it to make it last a long time on the shelf in the store. In the restaurant industry it is a huge rule that you don't slice more than you can use by today or tomorrow, to avoid waste.

Miriam came up with a way to avoid all the crazy chemicals in the sliced meat.

Problem solved.

Bake a whole turkey, pull the meat, leave out all the crazy nitrates, other fillers, and goop and only serve the real bird. It was a huge success with our customers and we avoided the crazy salt lick that is processed turkey!

Kristi: One of the best things about cooking a whole turkey is that you can use the leftovers in so many different ways. You can do a turkey and avocado wrap a turkey frittata and turkey and pesto pizza, well I could go on!

Miriam: Oh those all sound delish, let's put those in the recipe section.

Kristi: Sounds Great! Those were so popular with our restaurant customers. I'm sure our readers would adore them as much as our customers.

Miriam: Stay tuned for scrumptious turkey recipes, later on in the book.

Kristi: Yes remember let us not think of turkey just for Thanksgiving, it can be cooked and eaten all year long. That reminds me of a story.

Miriam: We all love your stories.

True Story:

I went to spend Thanksgiving with some long lost relatives and a huge crowd of their friends. Everybody brought something like a potluck dinner. So all throughout the kitchen there were pots and dishes and casseroles of "items" I totally did NOT recognize.

Bits and bobs of browned "items" and mashed "whatchamacallits" and soups of "wonders". I searched and searched for the turkey. To the point the hostess finally said, "What is it you are searching for?" I said, in a kind of loud voice, trying to be funny, "I think the Turkey has run off I can't find it. Ha Ha."

There was a collective gasp from all the dinner guests, so powerful it sucked the tea towels off the counter. They all, in a perturbed unison answered, "We're Vegans!"

Miriam: EEK!

Kristi: Yeah. To make matters worse. I laughed and said, "What? Ha Ha... (Seeing the not too thrilled look on my cousins face, I continued by saying) Ha Ha Ha, kidding. I knew that would get your goat, I mean tofu!

Miriam: Did you know they have a vegan turkey now? It's called Tofurkey. Interesting.

Kristi: The spell check on the computer totally does not like that name Tofurkey!

The blinding deception we found at the grocery store.

They are now selling sliced turkey with added caramel coloring around the edges that is cut in odd shapes to make it look like someone cut the turkey by hand.

Miriam: I was surprised, I guess I shouldn't be surprised at the intentional deception. But I was surprised none the less to discover, they now have a patented slicer for cutting the deli "turkey" that will slice the "No Food meat" unevenly like you would if you were using a knife and carving it at home.

According to their research they found that people felt they were buying something healthier when they saw what appeared to be "hand carved" meat.

Kristi: That just chaps my hide.

Miriam: I know it is crazy that the research and the product are intentionally designed to mislead. But it's not the only product out there doing that.

 They are trying to give you the feel of turkey at Grandma's on Sunday afternoon.

Our question is how many more chemicals have to be in that "meat" that they sell that is already sliced, and it can still have a long shelf life after you open it?

Miriam: Also, the caramel coloring that they add to the edges is MSG. Doesn't sound like Grandma's Sunday turkey to me!

Salt is an Appetite Stimulant

Have you ever noticed when you eat something salty you need something sweet to follow it down? Then if you eat something sweet you immediately want something salty.

But what happens when you eat salty and sweet together? This is known as "sensory specific satiety."

It's when you eat salt and sugar combined, like salted caramels. Now your appetite for sweet is filled, but now you need the salt to balance it out. When you start eating the salt it is like a separate tank that now needs to be filled.

Since the salt and sugar are in the same food typically you will continue to eat the same food until it is gone.

Manufacturers caught on to this and started adding more sugar and salt to their foods so you would eat more. Example would be chocolate covered peanuts, usually we eat the whole bag but if it was just peanuts we would eat several handfuls and be done.

Tricky Trick

The manufacturers are now also adding fake sugar into the salt and sugar bloated foods so that they can appear to have decreased the sugar content. It is now sweeter with less sugar because the artificial sugar tricks your brain into thinking there is sugar in there.

But what really happens is that the artificial sugar makes you eat more because your body is searching for the sugar to hook up with the insulin that it already released.

So if you want sugar, have some dark chocolate or a medjool date or make a sweet shake.

Sweet Shake

1 frozen not super overripe banana

1 cup unsweetened almond milk

1-2 medjool dates (pits removed)

2 shakes of cinnamon

1/2 small avocado

Blend until fabulous. If I use the dates it really makes it very sweet the avocado will add a little fat to slow the sugar going into your system.

Back to the sugar/salt double whammy.

It sounds crazy, I know, but some breakfast cereals contain more salt than corn chips.

It's no wonder that after eating cereal for breakfast by the time we get to work we dive into the chocolate donuts that Wanda, everybody's favorite secretary, brings every day.

Then head over to the vending machine on break to grab a pack of peanut butter crackers.

What about our kids?

Did you know that 1–3 year olds should have no more than 1,000mg a day of sodium? 4–8 year olds should have no more than, 1200 mg of sodium a day.

Miriam/Kristi: That still sounds like too much.

An article from the Daily Mail from Jane Clarke says that it is not until a child is 11 years old that their body can tolerate adult levels of sodium.

1,000mg of sodium is 1/5 teaspoon of sodium that means children should have no more than 1/5 tsp to 1/2 tsp of sodium a day. You need to check out the sodium on the Lunchables and snack packs or Goldfish that most children consume by the handfuls?

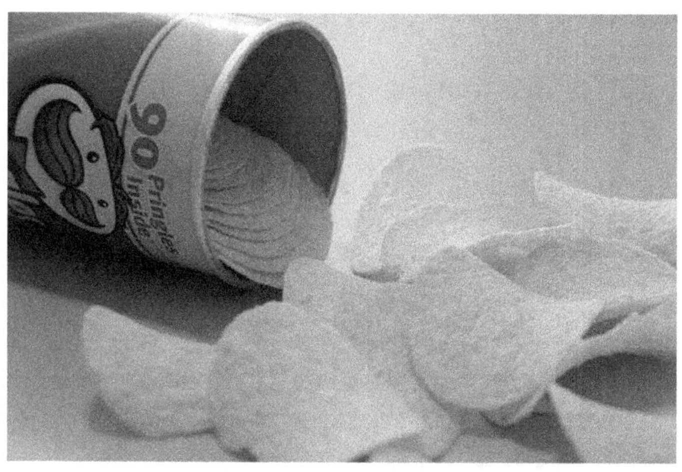

This is why our Kids are Fat

Peek Inside: Lays Sour Cream & Onion Chips

23 Ingredients MSG & salt listed more than once.

Potatoes, sunflower oil and/or corn oil, sour cream & onion seasoning (nonfat milk, less than 2% of the following: maltodextrin, onion powder, whey, salt, sour cream [cream, nonfat milk, cultures], dextrose, monosodium glutamate, palm oil, parsley, partially hydrogenated soybean and cottonseed oil, lactose, whey protein isolate, buttermilk, citric acid, natural and artificial flavors, lactic acid), and salt.

1 oz. of regular salted potato chips has 136 mg of sodium. A small snack size is usually slightly over 2 oz, so double the sodium.

1 cup of cheerios has 160 mg of sodium.

1 cup of Banana Nut cheerios has 200 mg of sodium.

1 cup of Special K is 204 mg of sodium.

Kristi: And who really eats just 1 cup of cereal? The way I use to eat cereal, eating just 1 cup wouldn't even be worth getting the milk out of the refrigerator! Cereal for me is like running with the Bulls in Pamplona. It lets all the "crazy making" loose, and I would eat half a box.

Miriam: We will have to talk more about stopping the "crazy making" in our next book.

Kristi: I want to tell our readers, that you are not alone. It is confusing enough to buy healthy foods, now you have to compete with the "mad scientist" manufacturers intentionally setting you up to fail.

For example. The reason the cereals don't taste salty is because the sugar that is in them fools the taste buds by detecting the sweet. The reason why chips taste saltier than cereal is because the salt is sprinkled on top and that hits the tongue first.

Remember we were talking about our kids snacks and grab and go lunches? Check out these facts.

Oscar Myers Lunchables Cheese Deep Dish has 500mg of sodium!

1 Armour jumbo hot dog 680 mg of Sodium.

Celeste Pizza for one 1,090mg of Sodium.

Giant Spaghetti Rings 970 mg of Sodium.

Ramen Noodles with vegetables 1,120mg of sodium.

Kristi: You know just the other day we spoke with a Mom that said all her child would eat was Ramen. I thought it was just college students that lived off Ramen. I know I lived off Ramen in college. If we were trying to be "Healthy" we would add a little frozen broccoli to the "Ramen".

Miriam: My how things have changed!

Kristi: I ate more than my share of Ramen noodles for dinner, and growing up I also ate more than my share of fried bologna and red hot dogs!

Miriam: We can all kinda follow that those aren't necessarily the healthiest dinner menu. But they make these little snacks so cute that you wouldn't think they were hiding something so unhealthy in something so cute.

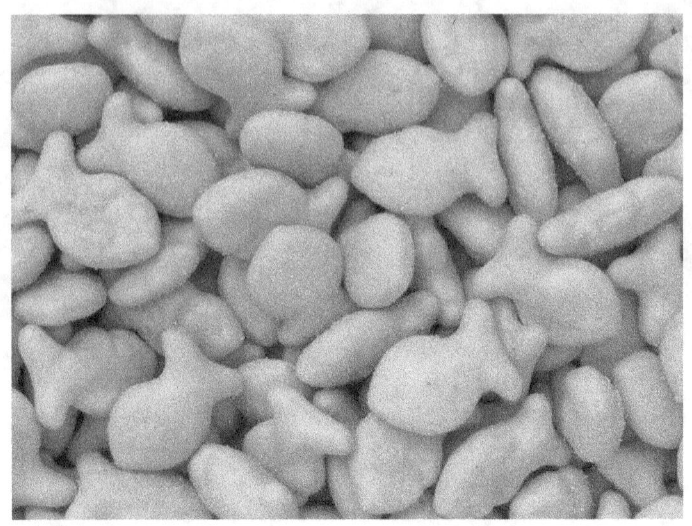

The Center for Science in the Public Interest, states:

Goldfish Cheddar crackers serving size is 55 crackers with 260 mg of sodium. For a toddler who will feed themselves out of the anti-spill snack cups that hold 110 crackers, that's 50% of their sodium intake for one day.

Of course we all know that they will eat more than one of those cups in a day!

Wouldn't it be just as easy to cut up pieces of apple or peaches and little pieces of grapes and pop those in the little cup?

Recap:

Convenience foods are only convenient for the manufacturers.

Want to be Fat? Want your kids to be Fat? Keep eating the "No Food" Food.

Deli meat has less protein, therefore it has less meat, than turkey from an actual turkey.

The more "Food Food" you eat the less tempting the "No Food" will be and you will lose weight because you will eat less.

"No Food" Food is cheap because it's not Food.

Healthy food is NOT expensive because you eat less and you actually get Food in your Food.

When your body has some real food to digest it will take longer so you feel full longer. Versus something that is nothing but chemicals and you are hungry in 10 minutes.

It's better to eat an organic apple and peanut butter and be full for a couple of hours, than a packet of nabisco peanut butter crackers and be hungry before you leave the parking lot.

I've eaten a ton of those crackers and 20 minutes later I'm asking Miriam, "Did we eat already?"

Chapter 5

Is Salt Making Your Kid Fat?

In this Chapter we will uncover the
"Foundation of Fat."

If you are trying to squeeze into your favorite
jeans or your kids are trying to suck it up to fit
into last year's swim wear, you will be very
interested to know the answer to that
question.

We build our and our children's Foundation of
Fat, one bite at a time.

 It's not too late to lay a healthy foundation
for your family.

Too much hidden salt in your food makes you
FAT. Here's why: when you eat too much salt
your body retains water in a futile effort to
flush the salt out of your system.

It's futile because every meal we are fed is
slammed full of hidden chemical-ized salt.

 An average meal at a national restaurant
chain can cost you on average of over 3 days'
worth of salt in one dinner!

Now there's a salt bomb you never ordered. That's why you feel like you are going to explode after you eat.

What we are calling Chemical-ized Salt is all the compounds preservatives additives colors and flavors that are derived from various forms of Chemical-ized salt.

Kristi: As we talked about earlier, Miriam and I owned a restaurant in Florida for the last 20 years. We have seen a lot of families come into the restaurant and bring food for their kids to eat.

This is where, as parents, you lay the "Foundation of Fat" for your children

As the parents say, "they just won't eat anything but chicken nuggets." As hard as it is on you as a parent to feed your kids healthy choices and get them to eat it, it's going to get harder as they get older.

If you start your kids off with so much sodium and chemicals at such a young age you will predestine the children to crave more and more salt and other chemicals that are expertly made in labs to cause cravings.

You are laying the foundation of fat for your child, one cheeto, and one chicken nugget one blue yogurt at a time.

Miriam: We are already seeing the effects of all the processed sugar and chemicals and salt in the children's diets. They are now diagnosing children with adult onset diabetes.

Also the incidence of childhood high blood pressure and heart disease is on the rise. I read a study the other day on the cbsnews.com that said this is the first generation that will not outlive their parents.

In 1976 five percent of children in the U.S qualified as obese. Today it's 20% or one-in-five kids. ~ CBSnew.com

We must pause. We must put the Lunchables and pizza pockets down. We must stop laying the "Foundation of Fat", we must stop eating on the run and eating premade foods that have loads of chemical-ized salt.

Miriam: Even trickier now the food industry is starting a new program that is called "Facts on the Front".

In this program the companies are listing the nutritional facts on the front. Like fat and carbs. But the problem we can already see with this is, we think, an intentional move on the food industries part.

The problem is that now people will just get trained to look at the "Facts on the Front" and ignore reading the actual ingredients.

Kristi: So companies will be able to slip in more and more chemicals to make the food appear healthy.

Tip of the Day:

Buy food that doesn't come in boxes and bags.

Miriam: We travel a lot and see thousands of brands of products, so many of the companies put all the certifications all over the bag. They are earth friendly, fish friendly, they use fair trade, they recycle the bag, compostable, you name it they have a certification.

But what's inside the bag is pure chemicals. It won't hurt the earth, but it may put you 6 feet under the earth.

Recap:

The Health of our Family is under attack. Childhood obesity, diabetes and high blood pressure are no longer an "Old Age" problem.

It's not your fault. You are being set up to fail by the giant food manufacturers.

The Most Important thing you can do today is eat at home.

Stop building the "Foundation of Fat" for your family. Buy single ingredient foods.

Turkey sandwich? Cook a turkey. Want French Fries? Cut up some potatoes and fry them yourself.

Want cookies? Get out the flour and make some.

All the Food Network Stars make cooking look so complicated and something meant only for "Reality T.V" they have everyone convinced that cooking should be left to the Professionals.

Life is complicated enough. Feeding yourself shouldn't be.

Kristi: In our first cookbook, Shake, Splash and Eat! Shockingly Simple Recipes. Miriam and I share small recipes that were our customers at the restaurant favorite single serve meals. We give you meals that serve 1 or 2 people in 3, 5 or 7 minutes. These meals are easy on the go options for busy family outings and quick weeknight nosh.

You can find our first cookbook on our website www.vigoacuisine.com

Miriam: Although I feel like we have covered a lot of information in this book my hope is that it will inspire you to grab the change that is possible.

Embrace the future with a healthy optimistic outlook that every bite makes a difference. That just because you have always eaten a certain way or certain foods, know that we can show you easy techniques and healthy options.

Eating well today takes care of your body and later on your body will take care of you.

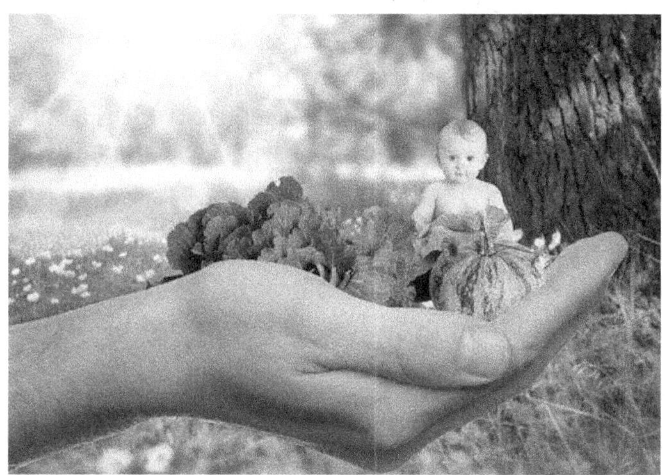

Chapter 6

Easy Recipes for the Busy Family

In this chapter we will share some very popular recipes from our restaurant.

When we retired from the restaurant we left many people having withdrawal from our flavors! So here are some simple ways to have that Shockingly Mouthwatering Restaurant Flavor you crave.

Our restaurant, as are our recipes, based on a 200 year old Family Tradition that Miriam recreated for our restaurant over 22 years ago when we first opened. She told us to Shake it up and Splash it on everything and everyone would go crazy.

Well they went crazy. It took our customers 7 years to talk Miriam into bottling her "Secret Sauces" so they could use them at home. The name of her secret sauce is Canary Island Garlic and Herb Olive Oil, we make 3 flavors Original Garlic Herb, Hot and Lime.

We still make them the traditional way from her family recipe in small batches. We use only Extra Virgin Olive Oil organic herbs and spices. We also put the day we made them instead of expiration date. We guarantee you will Love the ease of use and your family will adore the gourmet flavor.

Simply Shake, Splash and Eat! We give you restaurant flavor at home, without the work! These oils are Professional Grade Seasonings and are extremely concentrated. A little dab'll do ya.

Magic Flavor

One of the secrets of restaurant flavor, is proportional seasoning, what you want is the layers of flavor.

Layering flavors is the magic of successful restaurants. Every bite slightly different, the nuance of flavor every taste hits a different part of the mouth with a whisper of heat a kiss of lime or a splash of herby savoriness.

You want the Flavor of a restaurant in the comfort of your own home. You have found it.

We know you will enjoy the flavors and easy recipes that even our pickiest eaters can agree upon. So Shake, Splash and Eat!

-This olive oil is approved by picky eaters everywhere! (Joshua 12 year old picky eater)

Take good care: Miriam Vigoa and Kristi Linebaugh

Miriam's Famous Baked Turkey Recipe with Canary Island Garlic and Herb Olive Oil

Miriam: Here is my most popular baked turkey recipe it is so beautifully simple, it really can't get any easier than this.

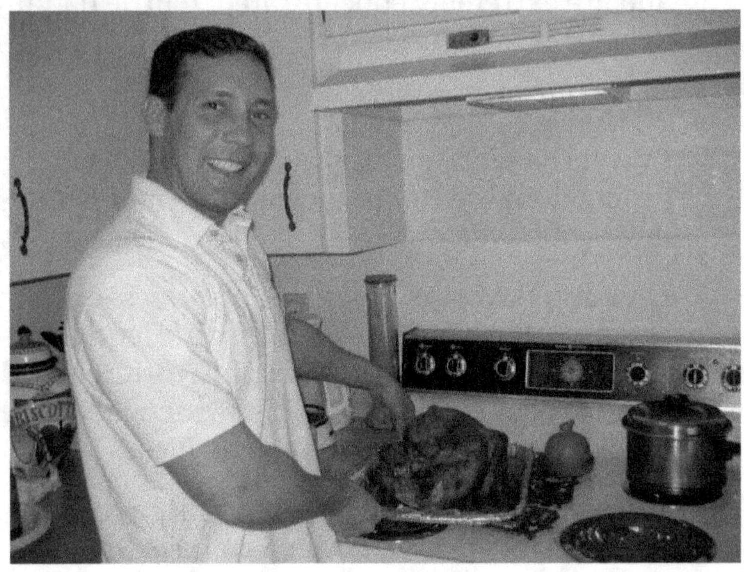

Kristi: I love this recipe, I can almost taste it right now. This is such a great picture of your nephew Father Richard Vigoa.

Miriam: Yes it is isn't it. I'm so proud of him. He loves sharing our family oils and cooking for friends.

Splash Turkey

1 20-22 lb Turkey

1/3 cup of Canary Island Garlic and Herb Olive Oil (The Splash),

Use your favorite flavor, Original, Lime or Hot

A.) Rub the turkey all over with the Canary Island Splash and put it in a baking bag, no need to flour the bag like the directions for the bag suggest.
B.) Follow all other directions on the bag. Bake till done.
C.) After the turkey is finished remove the bag and after it has cooled slightly, go ahead and pull the meat and put the meat in the juice and olive oil that was in the baking bag with the turkey.

If you leave the meat pulled you can mix the white and dark meat together and the combination of the juice and the Canary Island Olive Oil will make the white meat juicier and impart the most fabulous flavor to all the turkey dishes you make with it.

Bonus

Since the meat is already marinated all the recipes will have an added layer of flavor so if you freeze some of the cooked turkey, when you add it to stews or soups you will be delighted with the savoriness.

Be sure to freeze the meat in small portions so that you can grab a small bag and make one or two sandwiches without thawing a huge bag.

Kristi's Famous Turkey Avocado Wrap

This is a great way to mix and match veggies so if you like these veggies use them if you don't, use what you like and leave the rest.

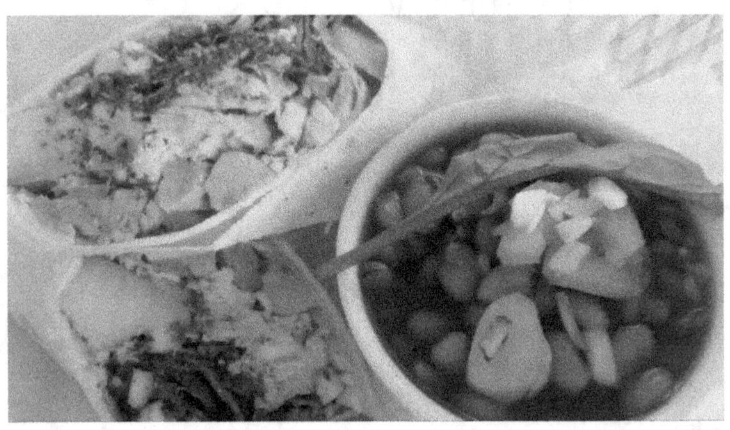

-These Flavors get your taste buds in an uproar!

(Joe Walsh, FL)

1 whole grain wrap

1 tablespoon cream cheese

1 4 finger pinch of baby spinach or arugula

1 ice cream scoop full of pulled turkey

3 slices of avocado, Haas avocado are smaller

1 Splash of Lime Canary Island Garlic Herb Olive Oil

1 Splash of Hot Canary Island Garlic Herb Olive Oil

1 Tablespoon chopped tomato and onion combined

   A.) Spread the cream cheese down the center and top with the spinach or arugula, then add the scoop of Turkey and drizzle the Lime Splash on Turkey.
   B.) Add the Avocado and the tomato and onion mix and drizzle the Hot over the rest.
   C.) On one side of tortilla add more cream cheese, tuck the ends in and roll the tortilla towards the cream cheese and use the cream cheese to seal the tortilla together. Cut in half and serve with a salad. You will Love Love Love it.

*4 finger pinch is when you take 4 fingers and grab a pinch of ingredients, 3 finger pinch is smaller and 2 finger pinch is smallest of all.

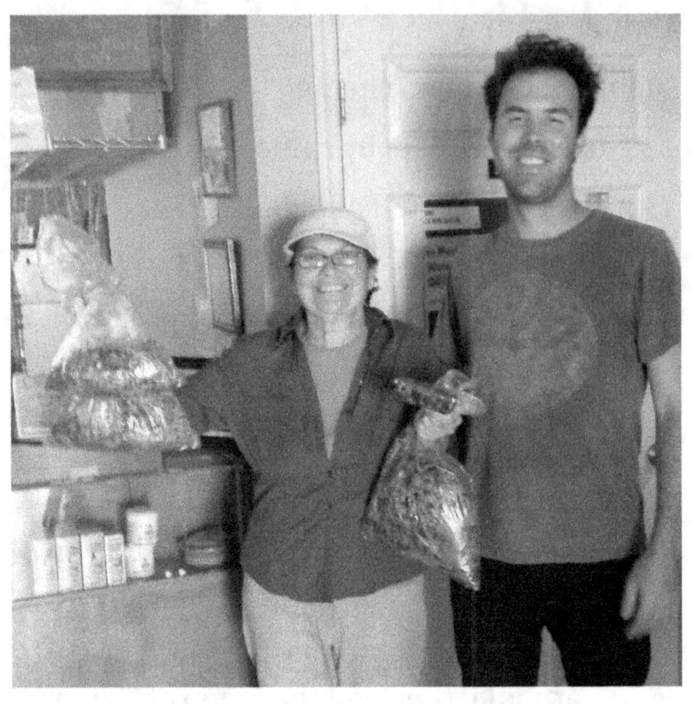

A great pic of Miriam and Will, he's from
www.CrumBrothersFamilyFarm.com. We
were his very first customer. He always had a
smile and of course the best arugula and
sprouts around!

Splashing up some Arugula Pesto

Pesto is easy to make in a small food
processor this is a recipe from the Food
Network that we reworked with the Splash.
Many times we get in a rut and think we can

use only basil in pesto but it is often hard to find fresh in quantity so using other favorite greens is easier to enjoy more often.

3 cups of arugula

1 cup parsley

1 garlic clove

¼ cup pine nuts or pecans if you like

¼ cup fresh grated parmesan (optional)

3–5 Tablespoons Original Canary Island Garlic Herb Olive Oil add a bit of water if too thick

A.) Turn on processor and drizzle the Canary Island Splash over the greens and nuts as they blend. If you want to leave out the cheese, use raw cashews in place of the cheese and the nuts.

B.) As the greens and the garlic and nuts blend, drizzle the Splash over till mixed. At end add the cheese and pulse several times to blend together.

Drizzle over pasta, sandwiches or grilled chicken.

"My Husband only has one kidney and is very restricted in his diet. Your oil is a Godsend for both of us!" (Mary G. WI.)

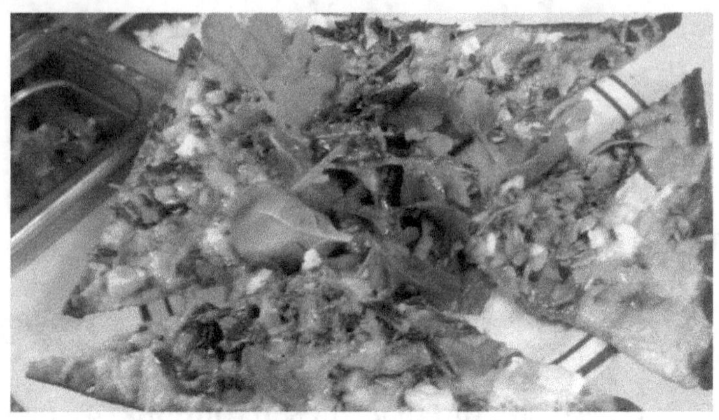

Zucchini Pesto Pizza

–I was overrun with zucchini in my garden this year and made this pizza repeatedly, but it was so much better with the Splash! (Renee, VA)

We didn't have a picture of Renee's Pizza so we used one of our own from the restaurant. You can see the prep board in the picture. Those tomatoes look so well organized!

1 wheat free crust from Udi's or Rudies

4 slices of fresh mozzarella

3 tablespoons pesto

1 thin sliced zucchini per pizza

1 tablespoon Original Canary Island Garlic Herb Olive Oil Splash

    A.) I drizzle Splash on the crust then top with cheese, zucchini and dollops of

pesto on top, followed by a drizzle more
Canary Island Splash.

B.) Put on grill for 5 minutes or put in
toaster oven for 5 minutes at 350-400.
Until crispy and cheese melted golden.

Bonus Recipe

You can also make these up ahead of time and
cut into finger appetizers and serve them
cold. If serving cold put the pesto on the
bottom with cheese then top with zucchini
that way when you are serving cold the
pesto is less messy when it's under the
cheese.

For our pizza we added thinly shredded
cheddar on top the mozzarella cheddar
combination is sublime.

Picky Kids Approved

"I give your oil a rating of 5 Thumbs Up!"

And I'm picky, just ask my Mom.

(Tabitha, 6 years old)

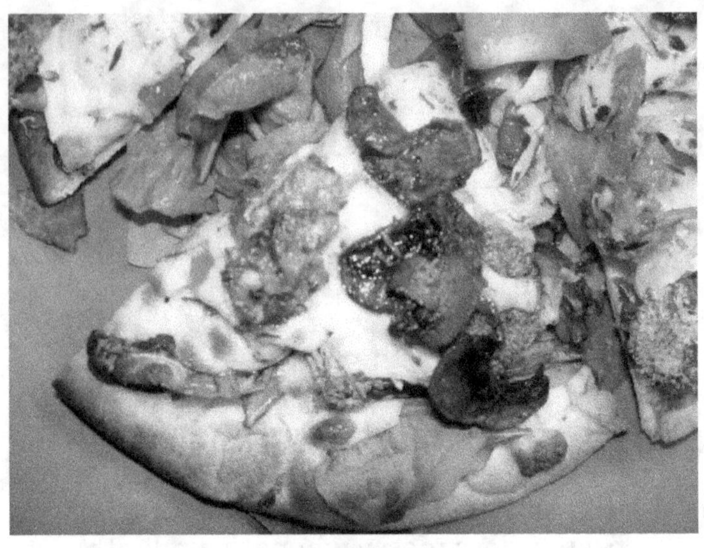

Spinach & Portobello Pizza
-I look forward all week to eating this pizza every Friday!

(Lou Belle, FL)

We served many healthy pizzas at our restaurant. We use to have groups of Weight Watchers come in to eat them because they were so low in points, but huge on flavor. We always tell our Weight Watchers, they can get Maximum Flavor with Minimum Oil when they use the Canary Island Garlic Herb Olive Oils.

1 whole grain pita (the kind with the pocket, not the gyro kind)

1 Tablespoon goat cheese (or cream cheese and feta)

1 4 finger pinch of organic baby greens or chopped watercress if you like a little peppery bite

1 3 finger pinch of sweet onion diced

1 3 finger pinch of zucchini sliced thin

1 3 finger pinch of red cabbage sliced thin

1 Tablespoon pesto dropped in 4 separate spots over the ingredients, add more if you wish

1 3 finger pinch of mozzarella you thinly grated

1 3 finger pinch of feta sprinkled over

1 4 finger pinch of chopped tomatoes

Sprinkle the already cooked baby portabello on top

    A.) Spread cheese over crust leaving ½ inch from outside crust. Add greens, and other ingredients in order listed.

    B.) Drizzle the Original Canary Island Garlic and Herb Olive Oil over the top from squeeze bottle. Equivalent of 1 teaspoon to 1 tablespoon whichever you prefer.

C.) Place in a toaster oven and put on toast
to simply melt the cheese and warm the
pita.

Bake it about 5 minutes in a toaster oven 350
is about right. As oven temperature and heat
can vary you may need a bit longer.

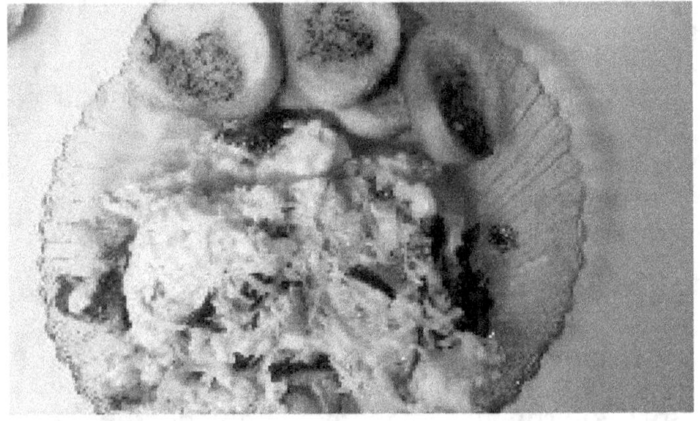

Veggie Frittata
A frittata is essentially an uncomplicated
omelet. For those not into complicated you
will love it.

2 Tablespoons Canary Island Garlic Herb Olive
Oil

1 3 finger pinch of chopped onions

3 cage free eggs

1 3 finger pinch of chopped baby spinach

1 3 finger pinch sliced zucchini

A.) Add the Canary Island Olive Oil to the pan and add the onions cook on medium 2 minutes then add veggies cook 1 minute more.

B.) Add the spinach and cook till turns bright green (merely seconds) and then add eggs to mix and cook till desired consistency.

C.) Optional, add fresh cold sliced tomatoes on top before serving and an additional splash of our olive oils.

For a nice change of pace you can also put all cooked ingredients into a wrap and then add it to the already hot pan and brown the wrap and serve that way.

Tip of the Day

Make these into the wrap form with leftover veggies and turkey or other protein with eggs while you are still cooking dinner.

Then after you make the wraps let them cool and put in the fridge and toast them up for breakfast in the morning. Better than burritos at McDonalds!

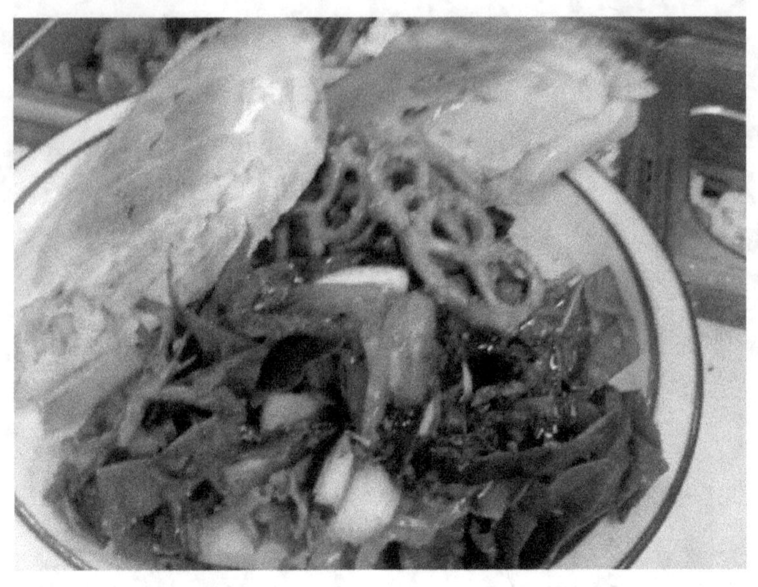

Grilled Turkey Cuban

This is a great alternative to a Cuban sandwich with pork. Our customers really loved these when Miriam would make them at our café.

1 8 inch piece of Cuban bread cut and opened like a book (leave the bread hinged)

3 sliced pickles dill kosher is good

1 ice cream scoop full of pulled turkey

1 3 finger pinch of fresh raw onions

1 drizzle of Canary Island Garlic Herb Olive Oils

A.) Place pickles then turkey on bread and
drizzle with Canary Island Olive Oil and
close bread and drizzle Olive Oil on top
of bread and put in Panini grill or pan
and press down to make like a Panini.

B.) After the bread is toasty and before you
serve add raw sweet onions on top of
turkey.

If you don't have Cuban bread French bread
will work as well, or if you have another
bread that is your favorite.

Drizzle our oils over the bread instead of
butter and grill like you would an old
fashioned grilled sandwich.

"Head over Heels"

*I love your olive oils, I've had acid reflux for years
and my sister fell Head over Heels with your oils
and brought them up to me in D.C. I'm so excited
to share it with my friends. When you find
something this healthy that alleviates that
"burning sensation" in my throat, I have to share
it!*

(Dottie, D.C)

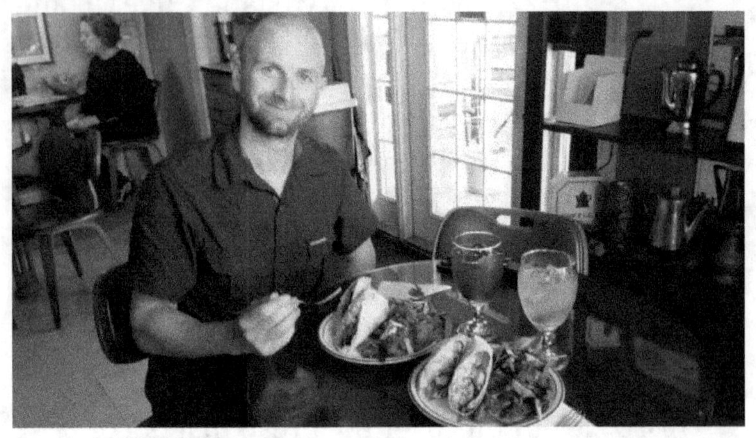

Stuart Bell getting ready to enjoy his Bangkok Boogie

Bangkok Boogie

Now this recipe is just for Tracy Eilers, she is one of our very first customers and she was with us all 20 years, she has asked for the recipe for years. So take Tracy's word for it. "It's the Best Wrap Ever!"

–Pleeeeze give me the recipe already! It's my favorite.   (Tracy FL.)

1 whole grain wrap

1 heaping tablespoon of plain hummus

¼ teaspoon red curry paste with lemongrass

3 finger pinch of organic baby greens

3 finger pinch of chopped thin zucchini or cucumber

2 finger pinch of shredded red cabbage

2 finger pinch of shredded carrots

3 finger pinch chopped tomatoes

6-8 golden raisins

1 tablespoon Lime **and** Hot Splash

3 finger pinch of shredded coconut

A.) Spread hummus down middle of tortilla add curry mix into hummus add drizzle of Hot Canary Island Olive Oil to hummus.

B.) Top with ingredients in order listed adding Lime Canary Island Olive Oil over top of coconut.

C.) Use dab cream cheese along side of wrap to stick together and put in toaster oven until wrap is golden brown.

Thanks for Splash–It's made the difference!

"Since changing to a healthy eating plan I put Splash on everything. If it wasn't for Splash I would never be able to stick to my plan!"
(Martha Santiago, FL)

Healthy Pizza Pockets

2 thumbs up from kids everywhere!

A big problem is getting kids and adults to eat leftovers. Here's a great way to repurpose your leftovers. After dinner if you have chicken and zucchini or hamburger and salad leftover. Turn them into pizza pockets.

1 whole grain tortilla or pocket pita in half

1 tablespoon of hummus or pesto or red sauce

Leftovers with mozzarella or feta

Stuff tortilla or pita with leftovers add your favorite flavor of Splash wrap in foil put in the fridge.

Or put the goodness on top of a salad, put in a Tupperware and take to work the next day.

Now you have either packed your kids lunch or you just made an after work, midday or late night healthy snack. Simply pop in toaster oven on a piece of foil toast till golden brown.

Having Withdrawal Symptoms

-I cannot be without this any longer. I've used it for 5 or 6 years and food isn't the same without it. I use the heck out of it, I've tried making it myself it is Not the same. I have to have it!
(Suzanne, GA)

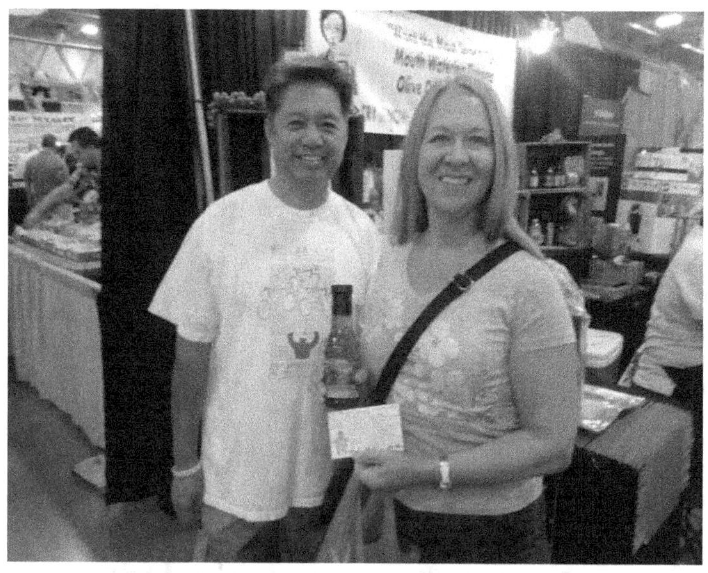

Grilled Pizza Recipe

Joan Crisostomo and her husband sent us this fabulous pizza recipe they invented and we wanted to share it with you. It's perfect for grilling season.

Use your favorite crust either fresh and bake it or premade crust, organic is best. Then cut up an assortment of veggies we love these but mix it up sometimes. Whatever we have. Heat grill to medium hot.

Eggplant

Mushroom

Red, yellow and orange bell peppers

Asparagus

> A.) Toss all cut up veggies with a few tablespoons of the Canary Island Garlic Herb Olive Oil and grill, a grilling basket with holes in it works the best.
> B.) Put a small of amount of the Canary Island Olive Oil on a grilling pan or use a cookie sheet so it won't stick, if you don't like the charred polka dots on the bottom of the pizza dough it's best to use a cookie sheet.
> C.) Add a small amount of red sauce to the dough and top with the roasted veggies, we also like to add shredded chicken and a bit more Canary Island to it.
> D.) Top with mozzarella and grill for 5-10 minutes or until crust is nice and golden toasty. Slice and Enjoy!

Bonus Recipe

In the morning take any leftover veggies and add a bit of the red sauce and reheat and serve it hot over your scrambled eggs as a ratatouille breakfast scramble add cheese if you are in the mood.

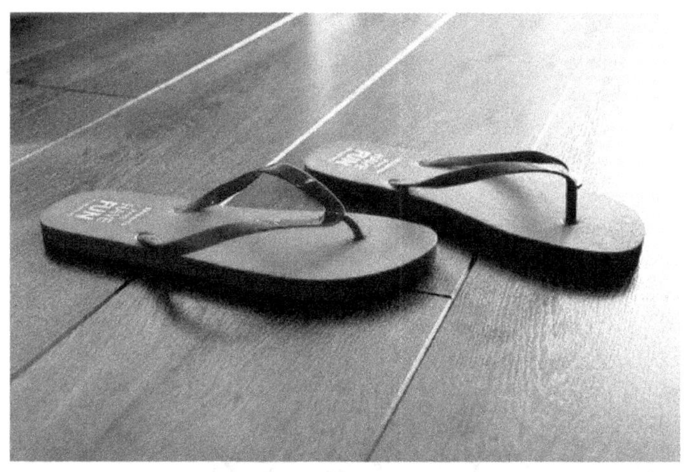

Flip Flops

*-This Dern oil is so good if you put it on a flip flop
I could eat it! (John, IN)*

:-) We are pretty proud, we use only the highest quality organic herbs and spices to make our fresh small batch seasoned olive oils. You can "Splash" them on everything without a worry of inflammation causing chemicals, weird oils or loads of salt and sugar. Canary Island Garlic Herb Olive Oil is 15 mg of sodium (10mg is considered salt free) and No sugar.

We use only Extra Virgin Olive Oil.

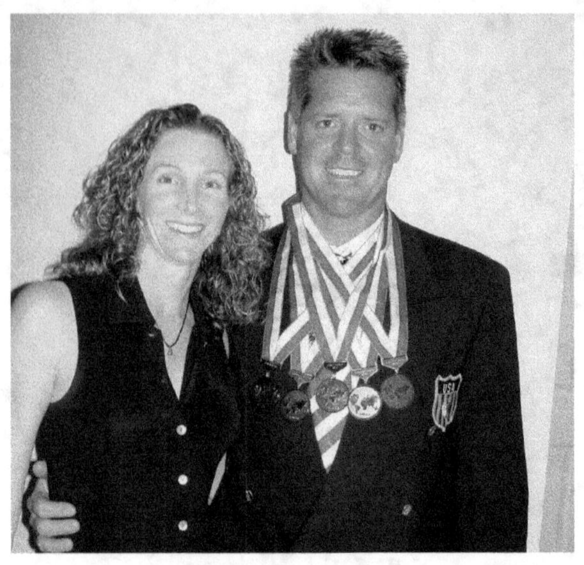

Cindy Bowers & Lane "Dawg" Bowers

Green Monster Protein Drink

This is my favorite drink from Café Latte it gets me pumped to push the envelope for an Amazing day on the water! Expect A Miracle!

www.TheFootersEdge.com

(Lane Bowers–2003 World Champion Barefoot Water Skier)

1 cup almond milk

1 handful organic baby spinach

1 tablespoon raisins

1 heaping tablespoon natural peanut butter

1 dash of cinnamon

1 scoop pea protein (optional)

1 cup ice

1 frozen banana (optional)

A.) Blend until silky smooth if too thick
add a bit more almond milk or cold
water, and sip your way into the day.
This drink is full of iron to help
oxygenate your blood so get ready for a
super duper day!

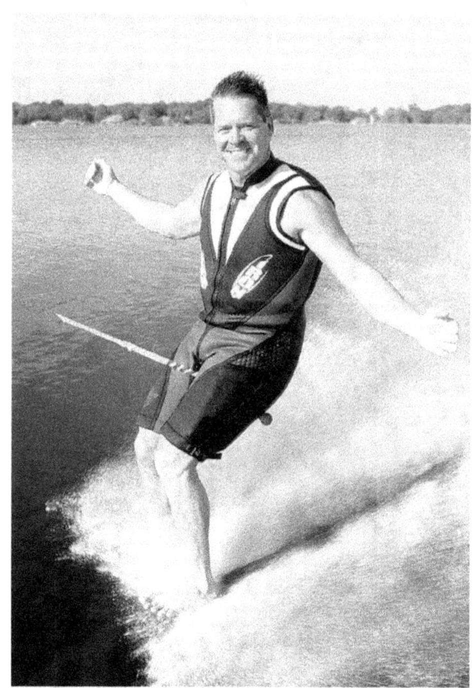

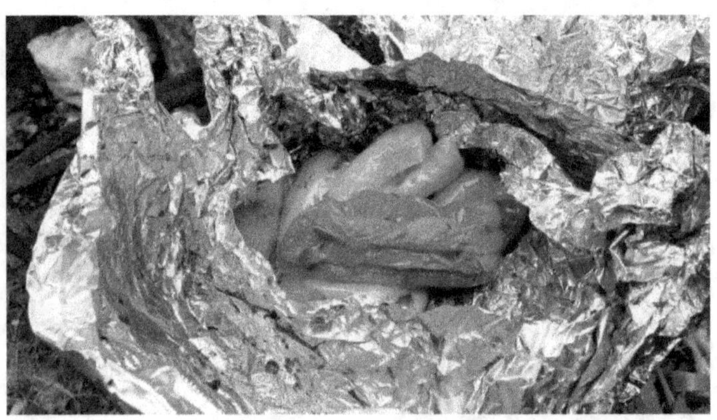

Miriam: This is a fun idea we did on a grill up in Michigan when we are on our Summer Tour we cook a lot at parks so we can grill our food and use the Splash to keep our chemicals out.

Kristi: I remember that picture we were on a lake and it was really windy and I was trying to wrap up the peppers and the foil kept flying away. I spent more time chasing foil than I did cooking!

Super Easy: 2 Tablespoons Hot Splash and 6 sweet peppers sliced and de-seeded 3 cloves of peeled garlic and wrap on throw in the back of the grill not directly over flame, flip after 10 minutes let sit another 5 to 10 minutes. Or go crazy and throw all type of veg in there!

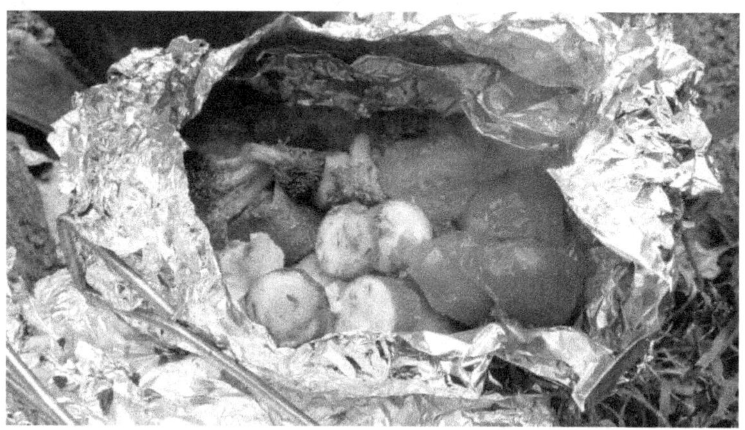

Splash Roasted Veggie Panini

Roasted veggies are easy to make once and enjoy all week. We use rutabaga, onions, peppers, carrots, celery, beets, acorn squash, fingerling potatoes, garlic cloves, zucchini or other veggies you adore.

    A.) Spread cut veggies onto cookie sheet and drizzle Canary Island Garlic Herb

Olive Oil over the top, don't drown them, just a nice drizzle.

B.) Oven on 400 for 20 minutes, using a spatula every five minutes scoop the veggies around flipping and mixing the olive oil over them as they bake. Or wrap in foil and throw on the grill for 10 minutes each side.

C.) For open face sandwich put hummus on bottom bread and top with favorite greens, arugula or sprouts and top with veggies and serve with a salad.

Bonus Recipe

Not in the mood for bread, make a big organic salad and drizzle the Canary Island Garlic and Herb Olive Oil with a little Braggs Apple Cider Vinegar over the top and scoop hummus in the middle of salad and top with the roasted veggies.

Then a teeny weeny little drizzle of honey over the top of the veggies and sprinkle your favorite nuts over the salad and some cut up fresh apples or pears.

My friend made me do it!

–My friend brought me to your booth the first time and said if you don't buy (Canary Island Garlic Herb Olive Oil) for yourself I'll buy it for you! I'm so glad she did, I love this stuff, now I'm hooked too! (Susan, Chicago)

Dinner for Breakfast Wraps

Now make breakfast while making dinner. This is a big hit with busy families also it's easy for kids to pop in the toaster oven for a hearty hand held breakfast.

While cooking dinner, make extra veggies and a bit of the meat you are to serve and before dinner just put meat and veggies and chopped greens in a pan and add 3-5 eggs and scramble together.

Use one ice cream scooper full of hot ingredients and wrap them in a tortilla and set out to cool while you eat dinner.

After dinner is over simply wrap in foil and put in fridge healthy done during dinner.

Now breakfast is ready or shoot it even works for lunch just pop in your lunch sack and reheat at work!

Personal Note:

We want to end this edition of the book with a quick update. There has been such an outpouring of interest in Kristi's weight loss (35 lbs. in 3 months) making it a total of 50 lbs. since incorporating my system called "Fresh Plates," all total she has lost 70lbs and she has kept it off for 3 years.

 We have been asked to share the techniques and tips we developed. So keep your eyes peeled we are currently working on our third book which will break down the easy steps to her life changing weight loss.

Miriam: Well this has been great fun! We'll have to do this again.

Kristi: Yes, definitely. Thank you guys for checking out our book we look forward to keeping in touch so be sure to stick around. We appreciate you!

Take good care,

Miriam Vigoa and Kristi Linebaugh

www.facebook.com/vigoacuisine

www.instagram.com/canaryislandoliveoil

www.twitter.com/kristilinebaugh

www.twitter.com/miriamvigoa

Interested in purchasing Canary Island Garlic Herb Olive Oils?

Whenever you are ready here are 6 more ways we can help you.

You may purchase our oil at the following new locations.

Lucky's Markets in Florida

Whole Foods Markets in Florida

Anna Maria Olive Oil Outpost

Rutabagas Health Food Store (Inverness, FL.)

Food for Thought (Sebring, FL.)

Health Food Center of Winter Haven, FL.

Amazon

ETSY www.vigoacuisine.etsy.com

www.vigoacuisine.com

Always remember we are old school as well so you can always just give us a jingle on the telephone.

800.975.2677

Miriam@vigoacuisine.com

Kristi@vigoacuisine.com

Our first and second book are now available on Amazon.

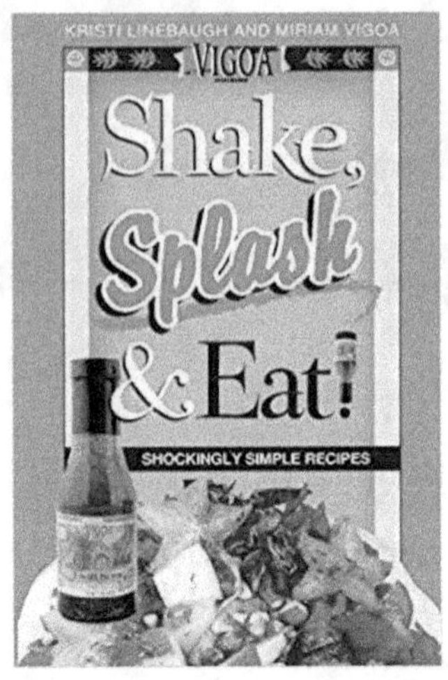

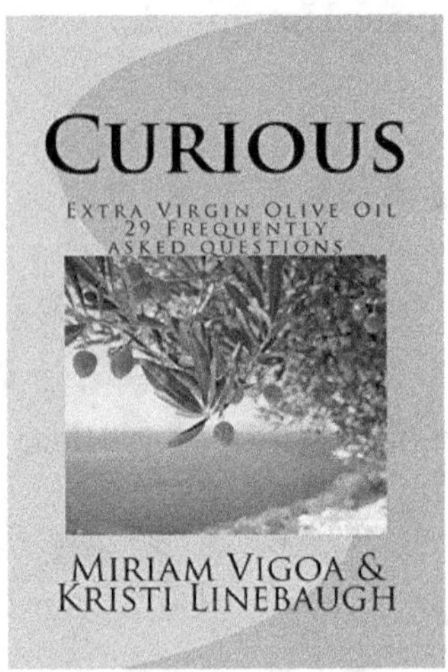

Take good care, we will see you soon!

Miriam Vigoa and Kristi Linebaugh